MENOPAUSE

MENOPAUSE

Derek Llewellyn-Jones
and
Suzanne Abraham

ASHWOOD HOUSE/PENGUIN BOOKS

Penguin Books Australia Ltd
487 Maroondah Highway, P.O. Box 257
Ringwood, Victoria, 3134, Australia
Penguin Books Ltd
Harmondsworth, Middlesex, England
Viking Penguin Inc.
40 West 23rd Street, New York, N.Y. 10010, U.S.A.
Penguin Books Canada Limited
2801 John Street, Markham, Ontario, Canada, L3R IB4
Penguin Books (N.Z.) Ltd
182–190 Wairau Road, Auckland 10, New Zealand

First published by Penguin Books Australia, 1988

Created and produced by Ashwood House Publishers
Typeset in Caslon and Avant Garde
by Abb-typesetting Pty. Ltd., Melbourne, Australia
Made and printed in Australia by The Book Printer, Blackburn

Llewellyn-Jones, Derek, 1923–
Menopause

Bibliography
Includes index
ISBN 014 011719 9

1. Menopause — Popular works. I. Abraham, Suzanne.
11. Title

618.1'75

CONTENTS

1 MENOPAUSE — AN INTRODUCTION   1

2 A WOMAN'S REPRODUCTIVE ORGANS   5

3 MENSTRUATION AND THE MENOPAUSE   14

4 PSYCHOLOGICAL CHANGES DURING THE
MENOPAUSE   23

5 THE PHYSICAL SYMPTOMS OF THE MENOPAUSE   27

6 HOW TO MANAGE THE MENOPAUSE   34

7 THE SIDE-EFFECTS OF HORMONAL TREATMENT   60

8 A HEALTHY DIET FOR THE MENOPAUSE
AND AFTER   65

9 OSTEOPOROSIS   76

10 THE MENOPAUSE AND BODY SYSTEMS   98

11 THE MENOPAUSE AND THE SKIN   112

12 THE MENOPAUSE AND THE MIND   120

13 THE MENOPAUSE AND SEXUALITY   129

   BIBLIOGRAPHY   133

   GLOSSARY   141

   INDEX   143

1

MENOPAUSE — AN INTRODUCTION

In biological terms, a woman's life may be divided into three overlapping periods. The first is childhood and early adolescence, extending to about the age of 15. During this period the child's body grows and, after puberty, develops into the characteristic female shape. The changes occurring around puberty are hormonally induced, and have the function of enabling the woman to conceive and bear children. In other words, they enable her to enter the second period of her life, the reproductive years.

The reproductive years extend to about the age of 50. Between the ages of 18 to 40, ovulation and menstruation occur more or less regularly at monthly intervals, and the woman has the choice of whether or not she will try to become pregnant. From about the age of 40, subtle hormonal changes begin to occur. These changes reduce the woman's likelihood of becoming pregnant, may alter her menstrual pattern, and lead, inexorably, to the menopause. Menopause means the cessation of menstruation, but the term is used to define the years around that event, when certain hormones are altering in various ways. Climacteric or perimenopause are more correct terms for the years around the menopause, but are not used as frequently as the term 'menopause'.

Following the menopause, a woman enters the third biological period of her life, the postmenopausal years. This period can be as fulfilling as the earlier periods but in many Western societies it has been perceived in a negative manner. For example, take this quotation from a book written in France in

1850, and entitled *Hygiene Rules Relative to the Change of Life*.

> Compelled to yield to the power of time, women now cease to exist as the species, and henceforward live only for themselves. Their features are stamped with the impress of age, and their genital organs are sealed with the signet of sterility. The first advice they ought to receive is to reject all sorts of drugs and receipts that are loudly proclaimed by ignorance and puffed by charlatanism. They ought not to sleep upon feather beds, nor in any bed that is too soft and too warm, for such are attended with the disadvantage of exciting the generative organs, which should, henceforth, be left, as far as possible, in a state of inaction.
> It is the dictate of prudence to avoid all such circumstances as might awaken any erotic thoughts in the mind, such as the spectacle of lascivious figures and the reading of passionate novels.

The author of this negative view was, of course, a man! Society's negative view of the menopause and of postmenopausal women may influence the way a woman adjusts to the event.

In the United States, several investigations have been made to find out about women's attitudes towards the menopause. The more recent studies, using a short questionnaire, show that women have a wide range of attitudes towards the menopause. The better educated the woman, the less does she perceive the menopause as a medical condition. Among those women who perceived the menopause as a medical condition and a period when help might be needed, opinion was divided about whether hormone treatment was also needed.

Fewer than 10 per cent of American women believed that the menopause made a woman feel less feminine, or that men saw menopausal women as less desirable.

Several societies in the developing world reward women who reach the menopause. Among certain castes in Rajhastan, women look forward to the menopause with pleasure. With the cessation of menstruation they emerge from Purdah, can move around at will, can talk and joke with men, and acquire a higher status. Similar changes occur for Arabian women, who are restricted to being only with other women in their reproductive years, but can join in social life with men once they have reached the menopause.

Other cultures in Ethiopia, sub-Saharan Africa and Micronesia also respect menopausal women and give them a high social status. Women who live in societies where age is venerated, where grandmothers have a significant role to play in the extended family, where kinship ties are strong, and where menstruation is encompassed with strong prohibitions and taboos, welcome the menopause as a beneficial event, and do not dread it as 'the end of life'.

This does not mean that women in these cultures have no symptoms, which in the West are attributed to the menopause. Over half of the women experience hot flushes or sweats, and some experience other less well defined symptoms.

These isolated observations do not give a clear picture of the significance of the menopause to women in most developing nations, nor is there any information whether the women have menopausal symptoms as severe as those that many Western women describe. If they do have similar symptoms, how do these affect their lives and their relationships with their husbands and children?

This information would be of great importance to the 300 million women aged 45 or more who live in the developing countries of the world.

THE AGE OF MENOPAUSE

In contrast to the onset of menstruation (the menarche), the age of which has declined from about 17 years in the early 19th century to 13 years today, the age of menopause does not seem to have altered over the centuries. In all countries studied, among women of all social classes, whether married or single, childless or having had a large family, half of all women will have ceased to menstruate by the age of 50, and by the age of 56 nearly all women will have reached the menopause. It is normal for some women to reach menopause by the age of 45 or as late as 55 years. If menopause occurs before the age of 45 or after the age of 55, investigation may be advisable.

PREMATURE MENOPAUSE

A few women cease to menstruate before they reach their 40th birthday and are described as having a premature menopause. The cause of the cessation of menstruation and the hormonal changes that occur are due to the sudden, spontaneous disappearance of the egg cells (primary follicles) in the ovaries. The cause of the disappearance remains a mystery.

The woman usually suffers from hot flushes and, later, a painful vagina. She also has an increased risk of developing osteoporosis.

ARTIFICIAL MENOPAUSE

This is the term given to women who, for various reasons, have their ovaries removed surgically or irradiated, so that the follicles are destroyed. Once again they tend to develop more severe menopausal symptoms and a greater risk of developing osteoporosis than women undergoing a natural menopause.

★   ★   ★

In this book we look at the menopause from a woman's viewpoint, from a doctor's viewpoint and from a psychologist's viewpoint. Although these three perceptions of the menopause have much in common, a different emphasis is placed on this period of life by each of them.

We believe that women in the years around the menopause will be better provided for if they understand the hormonal, physical and emotional changes that occur. We believe it important for women to be able to talk with health professionals (and other informed women) about their problems, and to receive help from the health professional. The process is called counselling.

We also believe that certain menopausal symptoms are relieved by the use of appropriate drugs, especially the female sex hormones, oestrogens and progestogens.

2

A WOMAN'S REPRODUCTIVE ORGANS

It is rather surprising that many women reaching the menopause lack the knowledge of the organs that are found only in women — their genital organs. In a way this is understandable as many women are embarrassed about 'down there'. So embarrassed in fact that many women have never looked 'down there', using a hand mirror. Women are prepared to look at other parts of their body, but their external genital organs, the only part of their genital system they can see, are ignored.

Knowledge about the shape of a woman's internal organs and their function is the basis for understanding part of the process that goes on in the years around the menopause. For this reason, a description of a woman's genital organs is given in this chapter.

THE EXTERNAL GENITAL ORGANS

The anatomical name for the area of the external genitalia in the female is the vulva. It is made up of several structures that surround the entrance to the vagina, each of which has its own separate function (Fig. 2.1). The labia majora (or the large lips of the vagina) are two large folds of skin, which contain sweat glands and hair follicles embedded in fat. The size of the labia majora varies considerably. In infancy and old age they are small, and the fat is not present; in the reproductive years, between puberty and the menopause, they are well filled with

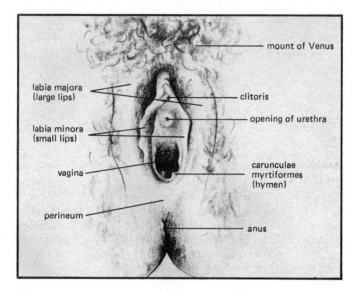

Figure 2.1: The external genitals in a woman who has had a child

fatty tissue. Looked at from between the legs, they join together in the pad of fat that surmounts the pelvic bone, and was called the 'mount of Venus' (mons veneris) by the ancient anatomists, when they noted that it was most developed in the reproductive years. Both of the labia, and more particularly the mons veneris, are covered with hair, the quantity of which varies from woman to woman. The pubic hair on the abdominal side of the mons veneris terminates in a straight line, while in the male the hair stretches upwards in an inverted 'V' to reach the umbilicus.

The inner surfaces of the labia majora are free from hair, and are separated by a small groove from the thin labia minora, which guard the entrance to the vagina.

The labia minora (the small lips) are delicate folds of skin, which contain little fatty tissue. They vary in size, and it was once believed that large labia minora were due to masturbation, which at that time was considered evil. It is now known that this is nonsense. In front, the labia minora divide into two folds, one of which passes over, and the other under the clitoris, and at the back they join to form the fourchette, which is always torn during childbirth. In the reproductive years, the labia minora are hidden by the enlarged labia majora, but in childhood and old age the labia minora appear more prominent because the labia majora are relatively small.

The clitoris is the exact female equivalent of the male penis. The fold of the labia minora that passes over it is equivalent to the male foreskin (prepuce). It is called the 'hood' and it covers and protects the sensitive end (or glans) of the clitoris. The fold of skin that passes under the clitoris is the equivalent of the small band of tissue that joins the pink glans of the penis to the skin that covers it, and is called the frenulum.

The clitoris is made up of tissue that fills with blood during sexual excitement. The end of the clitoris is often very sensitive to touch, but the area along the shaft of the clitoris, if stimulated, produces sexual arousal in the same way that a man is sexually aroused when the shaft of his penis is stimulated. In sexual intercourse, the movement of the man's penis in the vagina indirectly stimulates the clitoris and can lead to the woman having an orgasm. Many women do not reach orgasm during sexual intercourse but have deeply satisfying orgasms if they masturbate their clitoral area with their own finger or hand, or if a sexual partner caresses the area with his finger or tongue. The clitoris varies considerably in size, but is usually that of a green pea; as sexual excitement mounts, the clitoris increases in size. Once again, this varies considerably between individuals.

The cleft below the clitoris and between the labia minora is called the vestibule (or entrance). Just below the clitoris is the external opening of that part of the urinary tract (the urethra) that connects the bladder to the outside world. In old age, the urethral orifice may stretch and the lining of the lower part of the urethra may be exposed.

Below the external orifice is the hymen, which surrounds the vaginal orifice. The hymen is a thin incomplete fold of membrane, with one or more apertures in it. It varies considerably in shape and in elasticity, but is generally stretched or torn during the first attempt at sexual intercourse. The tearing may be followed by a minute amount of bleeding. In many cultures the rupture of the hymen (also called the maidenhead) and the consequent bleed is considered a sign that the girl was a virgin at the time of marriage; the bed is inspected on the morning after the first night of the honeymoon for evidence of blood. Although an intact hymen is considered a sign of virginity, it is not a reliable sign, as in some cases sexual intercourse fails to cause a tear and in others the hymen may have been torn previously by exploring fingers, either of the girl herself or of her sexual partner. Childbirth causes a greater tearing of the hymen, and after delivery only a few tags remain. Just outside the hymen, still within the vestibule but deep beneath the skin, are two collections of erectile tissues that fill with blood during sexual arousal. Deep in the backward part of the vestibule are two pea-sized glands, which secrete fluid during sexual arousal and moisten the entrance to the vagina, so that the penis may more readily enter it without discomfort. These glands, known as Bartholin's glands, occasionally become infected.

The area of the vulva between the posterior fourchette and the anus, and the muscles that lie under the skin, form a pyramid shaped wedge of tissue separating the vagina and the rectum. It is called the perineum, and is of considerable importance in childbirth.

It is a matter of constant surprise to us that many women have never looked at their own, or any other woman's external genitals, and consequently are concerned that they may be abnormal. We would agree that the diagram on page 6 is idealized to some extent and that a considerable range of shapes and sizes of the labia minora, the hymen and the hood of the clitoris is usual; so that if a woman looks at her external genitals with a mirror and finds what she sees is not exactly like the diagram, particularly in the length and shape of the labia minora, she should not be alarmed.

This reluctance to look at one's own genitals is a feminine trait (after all, men constantly look at and touch their external genitals) and has its origin in the attitudes that many mothers gave their daughters about their genitals. These attitudes are that the external genitals are 'private', ugly, should never be touched or 'played with', have a smell, and are 'dirty'.

Such indoctrination in childhood can have sad consequences to a woman's image of her own body and in her sexual response. Even the medical word for the external genitals of a woman is negatively loaded: it is the pudendum,

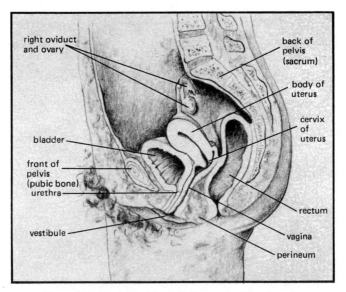

right oviduct
and ovary

back of
pelvis
(sacrum)

body of
uterus

cervix
of
uterus

bladder

front of
pelvis
(pubic bone)
urethra

rectum

vestibule

vagina

perineum

Figure 2.2: The internal genital organs of the female

which derives from the Latin word pudere — 'to be ashamed'. A woman should not be ashamed of or disgusted by her external genitals and should look at them to become familiar with their unique shape.

THE INTERNAL GENITAL ORGANS

The vagina   This is a muscular tube that stretches upwards and backwards from the vestibule to reach the uterus. As well as being muscular, it contains a well developed network of veins, which become distended in sexual arousal. Normally the walls of the vagina lie close together, the vagina being a potential cavity, which is distended by intravaginal tampons used during menstruation, by the penis during sexual intercourse, and in childbirth, when it stretches very considerably to permit the baby to be born. The vagina is about 9 cm (3¾ in.) long and at the upper end the cervix (or neck) of the uterus projects into it (Fig. 2.2). The vagina lies between the bladder in front and the rectum (or back passage) behind. At the sides it is surrounded and protected by the strong muscles of the floor of the pelvis. Unless the vagina has been damaged, injured or tightened at operation, or has not developed due to an absence of sex hormones, its size is quite adequate for sexual intercourse, and menopause usually does not influence this function. The vagina itself is a tube with an outer layer of muscle and an inner layer of cells.

The vagina is a remarkable organ. Not only is it capable of great distension, but it keeps itself clean. The cells that form its walls are 30 cells deep, lying on each other like the bricks of a house wall. In the reproductive years, the top layer of cells is constantly being shed into the vagina, where the cells are acted upon by a small bacillus that normally lives there, to produce lactic acid. The lactic acid kills any contaminating germs that may happen to get into the vagina. Because of this, 'cleansing' vaginal douches, so popular at one time in the United States, are unnecessary. In the years after the menopause, the lining tends to become thin, and few cells are shed, so little or no lactic acid is formed and contaminating germs may grow. This sometimes results in inflammation of the vagina, particularly in elderly women.

The uterus The uterus is an even more remarkable organ than the vagina. In the reproductive years, when the woman is not pregnant, it is pear shaped, averages 9 cm (3¾ in.) in length, 6 cm (2½ in.) in width at its widest point and weighs 60 g (2 oz.). The uterus is a muscular organ, located in the middle of the bony pelvis, and lying between the bladder in front and the bowel behind (Fig. 2.2). Its muscular front and back walls bulge into the cavity, which is normally narrow and slit-like, unless pregnancy occurs. Viewed from in front, the cavity is triangular and is lined with a special tissue made up of glands in a network of cells. This tissue is called the endometrium and it undergoes changes during each menstrual cycle. For descriptive purposes, the uterus is divided into an upper part, or body, and a lower portion, or cervix uteri. The word cervix means neck, so that the 'cervix uteri' means the neck of the womb. The cavity is narrow in the cervix, where it is called the cervical canal, widest in the body of the uterus and then narrow again towards the cornu (or horn), where the

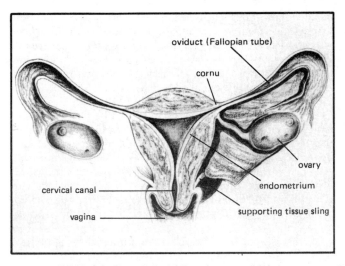

oviduct (Fallopian tube)

cornu

ovary

endometrium

cervical canal

supporting tissue sling

vagina

Figure 2.3: The cavity of the uterus, and tubes

cavity is continuous with the hollow Fallopian tube (Fig. 2.3). The cervix projects into the upper part of the vagina and is a particular place where cancer sometimes develops. The cancerous change in the cells of the cervix are preceded by alterations in their appearance, which may be seen when viewed through a microscope. If the alterations are detected, action can be taken to treat them so that cancer does not develop. This is the reason for recommending the examination of these cells by the Pap smear at regular intervals from when the woman is about 20 years old.

The lower part of the uterus and the upper part of the cervix are supported by a sling of special tissues, which stretch to the muscles of the pelvic wall in a fan-like manner. These supports may be stretched in childbirth, leading to a prolapse later in life. With better obstetrics and better education for childbirth, this complication is today much less likely to occur.

The uterus usually lies bent forward at an angle of 90° to the vagina, resting on the bladder. As the bladder fills it rotates backwards; as it empties the uterus falls forward again.

The oviducts   The oviducts (or Fallopian tubes) are two

small, hollow tubes, one on each side, which stretch for about 10 cm (4 in.) from the upper part of the uterus to lie in contact with the ovary on each side. Each tube is about the size of a drinking straw. The outer end of each oviduct is divided into long finger-like processes, and it is thought that these sweep up the egg when it is expelled from the ovary.

The ovaries In the reproductive years, the two ovaries are almond-shaped organs, averaging 3.5 cm (1½ in.) in length and 2 cm (¾ in.) in breadth. After the menopause, they decrease in size and in old age are less than half their adult size. Each ovary has a centre made up of small cells and a mesh of vessels. Surrounding this is the ovary proper, which contains about 200 000 egg cells lying in a cellular bed; outside this again, protecting the egg cells and the ovarian tissue, is a thickened layer of tissue. The ovaries are the equivalent of the male testes, and in addition to containing the egg cells on which all human life depends, the ovaries produce the female sex hormones during the reproductive years.

CHANGES AFTER THE MENOPAUSE

The tissues that make up a woman's genital organs are very responsive to the female sex hormones, oestrogen and progesterone. Oestrogen, which is produced in a woman's ovaries from puberty onwards, stimulates the growth of all the genital organs. This is why following puberty a woman's vagina grows and becomes moist, the uterus grows and menstruation starts, the Fallopian tubes become longer and thicker and the ovaries increase in size. The growth effect of oestrogen is modified by progesterone and a delicate relationship exists between the two hormones.

After the menopause very little progesterone is secreted and the level of oestrogen in the blood falls by at least 50 per cent. This is because the ovaries, having lost all their follicles, cease to produce oestrogen. However, oestrogen is still produced. This occurs because chemicals from another gland in the body, the adrenal gland, are converted into oestrogen in a woman's body fat. The quantity of oestrogen varies, depending principally on the quantities of fat in her body.

Over the years following menopause, a woman's genital organs become smaller. Her ovaries shrivel, each becoming the size of a small almond, and the Fallopian tubes become thin. Her uterus becomes small, in extreme old age often becoming no bigger than a thimble. Her vagina becomes narrower and its walls thinner. This may have two effects. The first is that the woman may develop a vaginal discomfort. The second is that sexual intercourse may become painful or impossible. The woman's vulva changes in appearance. The fat in her labia majora disappears, and her labia minora become more prominent. Slowly the vulva shrivels becoming a narrow dry slit in some old women. The changes may also affect a woman's bladder and may be a factor in some women of an increasing need to pass urine, especially at night, or of bladder infection. A few postmenopausal women find that they cannot control their urine, it dribbles out unexpectedly.

These changes occur at speeds that vary between women, and are halted or slowed if a woman either produces her own supply of oestrogen or takes oestrogen tablets.

A woman's breasts also respond readily to the stimulation of oestrogen. Many women observe that their breasts become fuller and more 'knotty' in the 2 weeks before menstruation. This is due to the effects of oestrogen. After the menopause the stimulating effect diminishes and the gland tissues in the breasts is reduced. Some postmenopausal women's breasts become small; in other women they become larger as more fat is deposited in them.

3

MENSTRUATION AND THE MENOPAUSE

During the reproductive years menstruation occurs regularly at reasonably predictable intervals. Most menstrual cycles, at least after the age of 16 and before the age of 45, are associated with ovulation, which occurs between 10 and 18 days before each menstruation starts whatever the length of the menstrual cycle.

Menstruation itself is the end of a complicated series of events. The ultimate controller of these events is a part of the brain called the hypothalamus, and even this part is affected by emotions and upsets. This is demonstrated by the fact that menstruation may cease after a particularly strong emotional upset. The absence of periods, which is called amenorrhoea, may persist for varying lengths of time. If the woman is not pregnant the periods usually return after 2 or 3 months; but in some women, amenorrhoea may persist for much longer. When this occurs, the woman usually visits a doctor. At this visit the doctor enquires about the woman's eating habits, her exercise patterns, and whether she has lost or gained weight. If the amenorrhoea has lasted for more than 9 months, the doctor usually takes blood to measure various hormones, as menstruation is regulated by them.

The sequence of hormonal events that precedes each monthly period is complicated and is more readily understood if one starts at the time of menstruation and traces what happens up to the time the next menstrual period occurs.

During the menstrual cycle, starting during menstruation, an area in the lowest part of the brain, the hypothalamus, releases quantities of a substance called gonadotrophin releasing hormone into the blood that supplies the pituitary gland. The hormone causes special cells in the pituitary gland to secrete a hormone called the follicle-stimulating hormone or FSH. The amount of FSH in the blood rises and stimulates the growth of 10 to 20 egg follicles. These follicles grow and as they do so they manufacture oestrogen, so that the amount of this special female sex hormone increases in the blood. Oestrogen has several effects on the tissues that make up the genital tract, but the one in which we are particularly interested is its action on the lining of the uterus. Oestrogen stimulates the lining to grow. At the end of the previous menstruation most of the lining had crumbled away and, mixed with blood and tissue fluid, had been shed as the menstrual flow. The lining is made up of narrow tubes, called endometrial glands, set in several layers of cells, called endometrial stromal cells. Oestrogen makes the glands grow, and the layers of stromal cells increase, or proliferate. Because of this, the changes in the uterus are called proliferative and this part of the cycle is called the proliferative phase of the menstrual cycle. As the follicles grow the amount of oestrogen in the blood continues to rise, and by 13 days after the onset of the previous menstruation, it has increased six-fold above the level found at the onset. The rising levels of oestrogen in the blood have an effect called a 'feed-back' on the hypothalamus, causing a change in gonadotrophin releasing hormone. The altered hormone is carried down the blood vessels that connect the hypothalamus to the pituitary gland, where certain specialized cells produce a substance called luteinizing hormone, or LH (Fig. 3.1). This hormone is so-called because it induces one of the egg follicles to burst and expel its contained egg, and it then changes the cells that make up the follicle to a bright yellow colour. (The Latin word for yellow is 'luteus' — hence the luteinizing, or yellow-making hormone). On about the 14th day after the onset of the previous menstrual period, a sudden surge of luteinizing hormone sweeps through the blood stream. It reaches the ovary, where it induces 'bursting' of the egg follicle that has grown the most, and that is blown up and tight like a tiny balloon. During growth this particular follicle had swollen and moved through the ovary to reach its surface, where it made a tiny bulge that can be seen by the naked eye. Suddenly, under the influence of the luteinizing

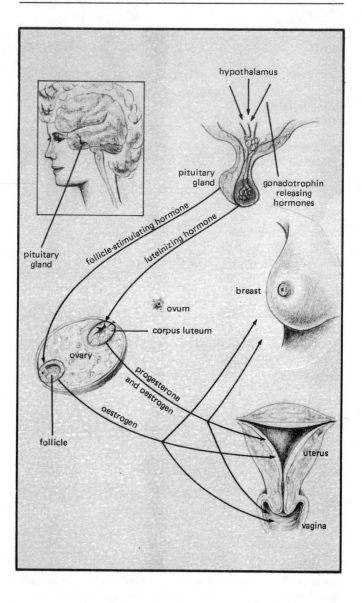

Figure 3.1: The control of menstruation

hormone, the follicle bursts and the egg is pushed out, together with the fluid in which it lay. The egg is caught in the finger-like ends of the oviduct, which caress the ovary at this time, and is moved slowly but gently into the cavity of the oviduct tube, where fertilization takes place, if this is to happen (Fig. 3.2).

Once the egg (ovum) has been expelled, the now empty follicle collapses, and the luteinizing hormone acts on the cells of its wall, turning them yellow. The collapsed follicle is called a yellow body or, in Latin, a corpus luteum. The change in colour of the cells of the corpus luteum is due to a change in their activity. Now not only do they continue to secrete oestrogen (together with the other 11 to 19 stimulated follicles that failed to grow as quickly), but uniquely they also manufacture a new hormone called progesterone. The name is apt, for the hormone prepares the uterus for pregnancy (progestos) — hence pro-gest-erone (-one indicates the kind of chemical substance).

Progesterone is the second main female sex hormone. It has

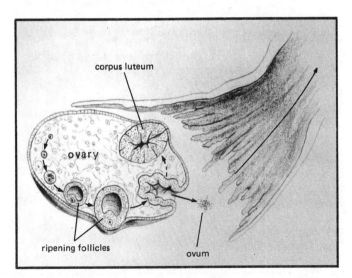

Figure 3.2: The growth of stimulated follicles in the ovary during a menstrual cycle

many actions, but the chief ones are that it relaxes smooth (involuntary) muscles; increases the production of the waxy secretions of the skin; and raises the temperature of the body. This is why it is normal for women in the second half of the menstrual cycle to have a temperature of up to 37.4°C (99.5°F). The part of the menstrual cycle after ovulation is called the luteal or the progestational phase. The most important progestational effect of progesterone is its action on the uterus. Progesterone thickens the lining of the uterus, and induces the glands to secrete a nutritious fluid and become succulent, so that a fertilized egg may be nourished during the time it needs to implant in the lining of the womb.

If the egg has not been fertilized and has not implanted into the endometrium, the yellow body in the ovary dies (as do the other stimulated follicles). When this happens, the level of oestrogen and progesterone in the blood falls. This has two effects: firstly, the restraint on the release of gonadotrophin releasing hormone by the hypothalamus is removed, and FSH production by the pituitary gland increases. Secondly, without the stimulation of oestrogen and progesterone, the now thick, juicy lining of the uterus begins to shrink and in doing so, kinks the tiny blood vessels that supply it. The kinked blood vessels (really blood capillaries) break, and patchy bleeding occurs in the deeper layers of the lining. This separates the lining above the blood; it crumbles and is shed into the uterine cavity, together with blood. Within a few hours, the amount of menstrual discharge in the uterine cavity is such that the uterus contracts, expelling it through the cervix into the vagina. Menstruation has begun.

Menstruation is the only visible demonstration of the hormonal relationships that occur in a woman's body each month. These relationships are important; if they are altered menstruation may become less or more frequent, heavier or lighter, last for longer or shorter periods and be painful or painless.

From the age of about 40, the precise interaction between the various hormones that 'control' menstruation begin to alter for reasons that are not yet understood. The most likely explanation is that the cells surrounding the follicles in the ovaries begin to become less receptive to the circulating pituitary hormones. In an effort to overcome the poor response, increasing amounts of FSH begin to be secreted, and the relative proportion of FSH and LH alters. This in turn leads to less frequent ovulation and, in some women, menstruation becomes irregular. As the years pass, the egg cells in the ovaries begin to disappear and their response to FSH is further reduced. In an attempt to stimulate the egg cells to grow, more FSH is secreted and its level in the blood rises, while a little later the level of LH also rises. Eventually, either all the egg cells disappear or most become unresponsive to the pituitary hormones, and the level of oestrogen secreted by them falls. The uterus is no longer stimulated and menstruation ceases. The woman has reached her menopause.

From this it follows that the menopause is associated with two major hormone changes. The first is that the level of the pituitary hormones FSH and LH becomes higher and the second is that the level of oestrogen becomes lower than during the reproductive years. Many of the symptoms of the menopause appear to be related to these hormonal changes.

HORMONAL CHANGES AFTER THE MENOPAUSE

After the menopause the levels of FSH and LH increase considerably (Fig. 3.3), while that of oestrogen falls. Oestrogen continues to be produced in varying amounts by postmenopausal women. The ovaries no longer produce oestrogen but continue to secrete substances from which oestrogen is made, as does one other organ in the body, the adrenal gland. These substances are converted into oestrogen in the fat that insulates the body. The more fat that covers a woman's body, the greater is the degree of conversion. The ovaries also produce the male hormone testosterone, as does the adrenal gland. The level of testosterone in the blood falls slightly after the menopause, but relative to the quantity of oestrogen rises somewhat. This may be a reason for the increased facial hair that occurs in some postmenopausal women. The blood levels of both oestrogen and testosterone fluctuate during the day and on different days, but the reason for these changes is not known. These fluctuations make it difficult, if not impossible, to relate hormone levels to the symptoms experienced by women in this period of life.

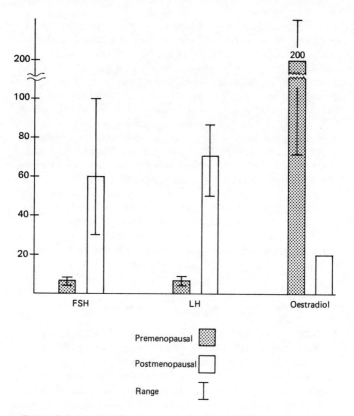

Figure 3.3: Levels of hormones in the blood in the years before and after menopause

WHY HAS THE MENOPAUSE BEEN LARGELY IGNORED BY DOCTORS?

Until 50 years ago, most doctors did not feel it was their responsibility to understand the problems a woman might encounter during the menopausal years. Most doctors perceived menopause as an event through which all women passed, which was not a 'disease', and for which no specific treatment was available. For these reasons menopause could be ignored or treated with sedatives. Such research as was undertaken was neither scientific nor rigorous. In the mid 1930s, with the realization that hormones controlled menstruation and that menopause was in some way due to hormonal changes, doctors became more interested in treating menopausal women, particularly as oestrogen could now be made in the laboratory. In the mid 1940s, oestrogen was selectively prescribed, but a dramatic change now occurred. Two American doctors advanced the opinion that it was every woman's right to be given oestrogen, and that failure to prescribe oestrogen was, in effect, medical negligence. Their argument was based on two doubtful suppositions. The first, as stated by one of the doctors, was that:

In 1900 the average life expectancy of women in the USA was 48.7 years. Sixty years later this figure has risen to 72.4 years. In other words, in half a century 24 years have been added to a woman's life, but the menopause still occurs at the same time. At the turn of the century Mrs Average launched her family and then died in her 40s, like a spent rocket, whilst today they have another 20 to 30 years of life.

The response to this supposition is as follows: in 1900, the *average* life expectancy at *birth* was low because many females died in childhood or young adulthood. Life expectancy at birth has increased by 24 years or so in the past century. However, if a woman reached the age of 50, her further life expectancy in 1900 was 22 years, while today it is only 6 years more (28 years). In other words, many women in 1900 did live into old age. But many children died from respiratory and gastro-intestinal infections, while young females died from tuberculosis or the effects of childbirth. These illnesses have largely been eliminated in the Western nations, so that many more people avoid the health hazards of childhood and young adulthood to reach menopausal years. In addition, because of environmental health measures and better medical treatment, the population is growing. This may be put in another way.

In 17th century Europe, about one woman in three survived childhood, adolescence and the reproductive years to reach menopause. Today, in the developed nations over 90 per cent of women reach menopause, and nearly all of them may expect to live until the age of 65. One in three women reaching 65 will live to celebrate her eightieth birthday. The effect of these factors is that although women reaching the age of 50 today only live on average 6 years longer than women born 100 years ago, there are many more postmenopausal women in the community.

The second argument goes like this:

Alone of the mammalian species, women live for many years after the end of their reproductive period. During these years they are deprived of the female sex hormones, particularly oestrogen, which leads to a variety of complaints. It is the right of every woman to be prescribed hormonal replacement therapy (HRT) to restore their bodies to health, vigor and beauty.

The retort to this argument will be discussed in a subsequent chapter. In summary it is not true. Not all women have menopausal symptoms, not all women have very low oestrogen levels; oestrogens have valuable effects when prescribed but they will not keep a woman 'forever youthful'. Further, although the post-reproductive years occupy about one-third of an average woman's life, post-reproductive years occupy the same *proportion* of time in monkeys, who live 30 years, and in rats, who live 30 months!

4

PSYCHOLOGICAL CHANGES DURING THE MENOPAUSE

The years around the menopause are a period of psychological transition. They are years when a woman no longer has menstrual periods each month, or episodes of heavy or irregular bleeding. After the menopause a woman no longer has to bother about contraception to avoid unwanted pregnancies. In a study we made of the attitudes of Australian women to the menopause, positive feelings were expressed by 30 per cent of the women.

Other women see the menopause in a less favourable way. Some women have to adjust to the fact that they can no longer bear a child. Others equate the cessation of menstruation with a loss of femininity, although few women express this view. Some women find the perimenopausal years are difficult because their children have become adults, have left home and have become independent, which the Americans call the 'the empty nest syndrome'. As the children may have moved some distance and are increasingly involved in their own relationships, some women may feel frustrated, angry, or experience anxiety or depression. If this occurs the woman may lose her self-esteem. Other women welcome the autonomy that the departure of the children and the cessation of menstruation provides.

During these years a menopausal woman may have to adjust to marital disharmony. Her husband or partner also may be undergoing a period of transition, as he adjusts to the loss of his dreams and the failure of his youthful ambitions. He may see his future in his job as unstimulating, uninteresting and stretching greyly for a decade or more. He may react to his problem by becoming obsessed with his work, or may become a fitness addict, or resort to alcohol as an escape. He may seek to get rid of his frustrations by 'taking it out' on his wife or by becoming utterly disinterested in her activities. The relationship between the couple may deteriorate so that minor disagreements become major wars. He may react to his confusion and concern about his future by forming a relationship with a younger woman, which tends to confirm his wife's belief that she has become unattractive, which she may blame on her menopause. In these ways the problems of one marriage partner become the problems of the other.

A menopausal woman may have to cope with other problems, which seem to become more serious because of her concern about the menopause. This concern is increased in a society that stresses youth. The woman may believe that the menopause signals 'the end of life' — at least of a life that offered challenges, joys, excitement, as well as dreariness and dissatisfaction.

The feelings of lost hopes, lost femininity, and a general feeling of confusion can be coped with in many ways. Some women cope splendidly on their own, others need a partner's support, often only solving their problems at the expense of the partner. Some women need help from others. Some succumb.

In general, women who have interests outside the home and domesticity cope better than women who only perceive their role in life as that of housewife and mother. Women with more financial, educational, social and cultural resources adjust better because they have more choices in life style at their disposal. In Sweden, at least, the women most affected are housewives with limited education and few interests outside their family. But these findings may not be applicable to women of other nationalities. Women who have a good relationship (including a good sexual relationship) with their partner adjust more easily than women who do not have such a relationship. Sexuality after the menopause is discussed in Chapter 13.

Single women also have problems in the menopausal years. Single women benefit by having a career and social interests, possibly to a greater extent than married women. But often they have no permanent partner to whom they can relate and with whom they can share their concerns. Although a single woman may avoid marital conflict, she may feel that the absence of children leaves her disadvantaged. The menopause is a clear signal to her that she will never have children. Usually a single woman has adapted, some years before she reaches the menopause, to her single status and to the absence of children so that she is no more likely to suffer psychological problems during the menopause than her married sister.

PSYCHOLOGICAL SYMPTOMS

It will be appreciated from what we have just written that psychological symptoms that occur in the menopausal years are not easy to identify. In addition, as we discuss in Chapter 12, the symptoms are not necessarily *due* to the menopause.

The most common symptoms reported in surveys of menopausal women are: an inability to cope with problems; anxiety; constant (or intermittent) tiredness; irritability and mild depression. But these symptoms are more common in younger and older women (see Chapter 12). In some women the psychological symptoms (at least as judged by recognized anxiety and depression scales) may be aggravated by life stresses. It also appears that the psychological symptoms, particularly anxiety, may exacerbate the physical symptoms such as hot flushes.

COPING WITH THE PSYCHOLOGICAL CHANGES

The importance of a helpful, supportive, understanding partner in helping a woman through the menopausal years is obvious from the previous discussion. However, in many instances the husband or partner is not equipped to help. A study in Britain in the 1970s showed that at least 25 per cent of the men were unaware of the nature or the extent of their wife's problems. Most of the men had no knowledge of the emotional changes that affect many menopausal women. Many husbands are unaware that a woman needs more love, understanding, encouragement and contact in the menopausal years. Many a husband is unaware that his behaviour may aggravate her emotional upset. The couple should start evaluating their relationship and trying to understand each other better. One way of doing this is to spend more time with each other, doing things that they both enjoy. It is also important that each partner learns to listen to what the other is saying and to talk *with* each other, rather than *at* each other.

Knowledge about the changes that are occurring during the menopausal years also helps the woman to adjust. This knowledge may be obtained from books, but for full effect books need to be supplemented by discussions in 'menopausal groups' or with an informed, empathetic doctor, nurse, clinical psychologist or social worker.

We write about the management of the menopause at greater length in Chapter 6.

5

THE PHYSICAL SYMPTOMS OF THE MENOPAUSE

A problem in identifying which symptoms are due to the reduced levels of the female sex hormone oestrogen and which are due to psychosocial changes is that doctors and psychologists have tended to look at the menopause differently. Doctors, in general, have seen the menopause as a medical condition due to a hormonal deficiency, which should be treated with drugs. Psychologists, on the other hand, have seen the menopause as a period of change, during which a woman has to adapt to and cope with a different role in life.

A few doctors and a few psychologists see menopause as a major transition into old age, or senescence. There is no evidence that the cessation of menstruation and the bodily changes consequent on lowered oestrogen levels is a marker of old age. Menopause is not 'the end of life'; it is only one of many factors demonstrating the ageing process.

However, if women in middle age are to be helped, it would be useful to know how many women have 'disturbing' symptoms during the years around the menopause, and what these symptoms are.

Here some problems arise. It is obvious, if you think about it, that doctors and psychologists who write papers for professional journals or who speak at meetings can only report on the people who have consulted them or have been surveyed by them. This may give other health professionals an unreal picture, as those people who are seen by a doctor or a psychologist may not be representative of the community in which they live, any more than patients who attend a cardiologist are representative of their community, or people visiting a

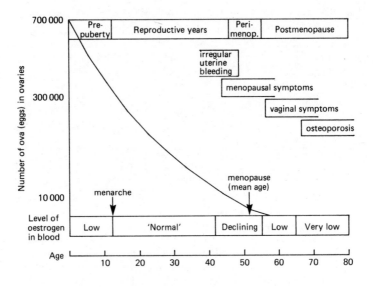

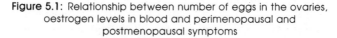

Figure 5.1: Relationship between number of eggs in the ovaries, oestrogen levels in blood and perimenopausal and postmenopausal symptoms

psychologist because of a behavioural problem, of their community. Because of this it is difficult to be sure how many women suffer unpleasant symptoms during the menopausal years. It is also difficult to be sure which of the symptoms are due to the hormonal changes of the menopause and which are coincidental.

MENSTRUAL DISTURBANCE BEFORE THE MENOPAUSE

Many women note that in their 40s their menstrual periods change. These changes precede the symptoms of the menopause, but like them are due to changes in hormone levels.

The main change is that the regular menstrual periods that have occurred during most of the woman's reproductive years become irregular. The interval from the first day of one menstruation to the next menstruation alters, often becoming shorter, occasionally longer or sometimes menstruation may occur at quite unpredictable intervals until they cease. These changes occur to about 35 per cent of women. Another 35 per cent of women may find that their menstrual periods occur at longer and longer intervals and then cease; and about 30 per cent of women menstruate regularly until the periods cease.

The quantity of menstrual discharge also varies between women; some women have scanty periods, in others the blood loss increases so that treatment is sought for heavy periods or for flooding.

In addition, some women start having hot flushes while still menstruating regularly, although in most women the hot flushes only occur when menstruation is irregular or after the menopause has been reached.

DISTURBING SYMPTOMS DURING THE MENOPAUSE

How many women develop disturbing symptoms in the menopausal years?

In recent years, anecdotal information has been replaced by community studies in an attempt to answer this question.

If the results of the studies are combined, it appears that in the countries of Northern Europe and North America, at least 75 per cent of women suffer some symptoms during the menopause and in one-quarter to one-half the symptoms are associated with physical or emotional discomfort. Of the 75 per cent of women who have symptoms, between one-third and one-half visit a doctor. The difference in the proportion of women visiting a doctor depends on how women in a particular community perceive the menopause, and on the influence on women of articles about menopause in magazines.

What symptoms are due to the menopause?

This question is harder to answer. This is because symptoms due to menopause may be confused with symptoms due to a change in the woman's life-style or to the ageing process. In past years doctors have tended to list symptoms as diverse as dryness of hair and aching toe-joints as caused by the menopause. However, these doctors were not as undiscriminating as an English doctor who wrote a book in 1870 entitled: *The Change of Life in Health and Disease*. In this book he listed

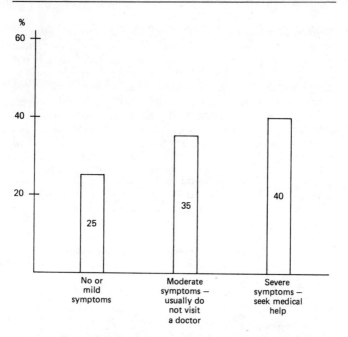

Figure 5.2: Severity of menopausal symptoms

135 conditions he ascribed to the menopause, ranging from temporary deafness through 'hysterical flatulence' to 'boils in the seat' and 'blind piles'!

Several investigators have tried to obtain more precise information about menopausal symptoms, but unfortunately the way they have done the investigations have made most of the results difficult to interpret. In 1980, an attempt was made to overcome this problem by a group of doctors in Oxfordshire, England. They asked a group of women and men aged 30 to 64 to complete two questionnaires. In all, 1120 women and 510 men were chosen by random sample with about equal numbers in each 5-year age group. The questionnaires were mailed at a 6-week interval asking questions about the person's health. No mention was made that menopausal symptoms were being investigated.

The survey showed that only two sets of symptoms were

associated with the menopause. These were hot flushings and night and day sweats. Two years later, two Swedish studies reported similar findings to those from Oxfordshire. The Swedish studies reported one additional group of symptoms associated with the years just after the menopause had been reached. They found that between 15 and 25 per cent of the women they studied complained of vaginal dryness or vaginal 'burning', which in some cases made intercourse painful or impossible. These symptoms only affected a few women in the early postmenopausal years, but the proportion increased as the women became older.

The English doctors found another matter of interest. This was that women aged 45 to 50, who usually had not reached their menopause, complained that they often had difficulty in making decisions and had a greater likelihood of having lost their confidence than younger or older women. These emotional changes might be due to hormonal changes but it is more likely that they are due to a negative cultural perception of menopause. This perception by society and by the woman herself may cause her to lose her belief in her value to herself and to others, and may cause her to lose her self confidence.

The studies from England and Sweden suggest that only two groups of symptoms are caused by the menopause. In the first group are the *vasomotor symptoms* of hot flushes, sweats and insomnia. The second group includes: *vaginal dryness, discomfort and sometimes burning.* The vaginal symptoms and painful intercourse that occur because of them usually are not severe until 5 or more years after the menopause.

The vasomotor symptoms

The majority of menopausal women who present to a doctor complain of hot flushes (called hot flashes in the USA). A hot flush has been described by one of our patients as follows:

At intervals I suddenly get a feeling of heat which starts either in my face and spreads to my neck and upper chest, or begins in my chest and spreads upwards. Occasionally my whole body feels hot. I know it only lasts for a minute or so, but it does disturb me. I keep waiting for the thing to come again. If it happens at night, as it often does, I wake up in a sweat. I throw off the bedclothes and often have to get out of bed and dry myself with a towel, then I can't get back to sleep again. In many of the flushes, I develop red blotches on my neck, and it looks ugly. When the flush finishes, I often feel cold, shiver a bit and feel stupidly weak for a short time. I have begun to hate myself and my flushes. I suppose that this self hate is making me more aware of my body, or something like that, because I now notice that sometimes my heart thumps and thumps and it never did before.

The frequency and severity of hot flushes vary between women. In many women the flushes are mild and infrequent and do not disturb the woman. In others they are so severe they may affect considerably a woman's enjoyment of life and her efficiency at work. Hot flushes precede the actual meno-pause in about 30 per cent of women (being more common when the periods become irregular) and persist for up to 5 years after menstruation ceases in 20 per cent of women. In most women, however, their duration is limited to about one year, starting at the menopause. About 40 per cent of women say that they have no flushes, in 20 per cent they are mild and in 40 per cent they are moderately or severely disturbing to the woman.

What causes hot flushes?

It is known that, following a brief 'warning', there is an increase in blood flow in the tissues beneath the skin and the pulse rate rises, but the blood pressure levels are unaltered. The episode lasts for 2 to 3 minutes, although the blood flow changes persist for longer, during which time sweating may occur. Flushes are associated with low levels of oestrogen but this cannot be the cause because the flushes usually cease in 1 or 2 years, while the level of oestrogen falls further as the woman grows older. But it is possible that during the transi-tional period of the early menopause, because of the fall in oestrogen levels in the blood, a woman's vascular system is 'made more sensitive to the effects of certain brain hormones and opium-like substances' so that it is less well controlled. This mechanism would account for the flushes, the sweats, the palpitations and perhaps headache, which some women say is more frequent in the years around the time menstruation ceases.

The dry painful vagina

One of our patients told us:

> The problem didn't start at my menopause which wasn't really a problem. But a few years later I noticed that my vagina felt dry and on some days I felt a burning feeling inside it. We don't have intercourse often now; my husband is older than me and doesn't seem to want it, but every so often he decides he wants to make love. That isn't really the right word; he's never really made love in recent years. No foreplay, just sex. Well, I accepted that but now I find that when he tries to go inside me it hurts. So I tell him to stop and he gets cranky. He doesn't talk to me for days until he's got over it. I suppose it is part of growing old.

Vaginal dryness, burning, and pain when the woman's husband tries to introduce his penis into her vagina, are symptoms that usually occur for the first time a few years after the menopause, but may occur earlier. Most women do not experience the symptoms, and when present, they vary in severity from woman to woman. They are more common among women who only have intercourse infrequently at long intervals. The cause is a thinning of the vaginal lining and a reduction in the blood flow to the vagina. You may recall that during the reproductive years the vagina is lined by a 'wall' of cells, 30 cells deep. The structure of the vaginal wall depends on oestrogen. After the menopause, with the fall in the level of oestrogen in the blood, the thickness of the vaginal wall decreases, so that it may be 10 cells thick or less. The acidity of the vagina also decreases, allowing more pathogenic bacteria to grow. A reduction in blood flow to the vagina aggravates the problem and the vagina becomes less able to distend. These factors — the reduction in the structures of the vagina and its reduced ability to expand easily — lead to the feeling of dryness and to painful intercourse.

6

HOW TO MANAGE THE MENOPAUSE

The menopause, as well as being a period of hormonal change, is a time of life-change, of renewal, when different aspirations are perceived and different challenges are experienced. For this reason the management of the menopause needs to take into account two interlinked but separate treatments. The first is psychological, the second pharmacological.

The purpose of psychological treatment (talking, psychotherapy or counselling) is to help the woman to understand her body and to become acquainted with the changes it is undergoing as she moves from the reproductive years of her life through the menopausal years into the postmenopausal period.

The purpose of pharmacological treatment is to prescribe hormones and other drugs to treat the menopausal symptoms for which they are specific. Hormone treatment is only appropriate for those symptoms that are related to hormone deficiency, which in most cases is a lack of oestrogen circulating in the woman's body. The two menopausal symptoms likely to respond to oestrogen treatment are the *vasomotor symptoms* of hot flushes, sweats and insomnia; and, usually later in the menopausal years, *vaginal symptoms* of dryness, burning and pain during intercourse. Some doctors and some women believe that oestrogen treatment reduces fatigue and increases sexual desire.

MANAGEMENT OF THE PSYCHOLOGICAL SYMPTOMS

Many of the symptoms both psychological and physical, experienced by a woman during the menopausal years are relieved if the woman takes into account her general health. During these years a woman may take the opportunity to assess herself and to look at her life-style, so that she can make changes that should result in a more relaxed, healthier and happier life. This approach reduces the impact of many of the symptoms that occur during these years.

Perhaps the most important action a woman can take is to understand what is happening to her body and to know what she may expect. We have found that many women feel that there is insufficient readily available information about the menopause. We also found that women perceived that many health professionals consulted were not particularly helpful, although individual doctors, psychologists or social workers were concerned and helpful.

When consulting a health professional, many women either do not ask about matters that concern them, or the health professional does not raise the issues. For example, women who recently have ceased to menstruate would like to know for how long they should carry a tampon in their handbag in case bleeding suddenly starts. As the menstrual pattern varies so much between individual women, this information is not available. Another question often raised by women is how long the hot flushes will continue, as a woman might be prepared to put up with the inconvenience without hormonal treatment if they only lasted for six months but would not if they persisted for 5 years. The reason that a woman wishes to avoid hormones may be because of the belief that the menopause is a natural event, or because of bad experiences when taking the 'Pill' earlier in life, or anxiety because the media usually only report sensational or adverse findings about hormones. Again, information about the duration of hot flushes in an individual woman is not available. Another matter of concern to many women is when the woman (or her husband or partner) can cease to use contraceptives and be sure that pregnancy will not occur. In our survey, 35 per cent of Australian women worried about pregnancy occurring during the menopausal years.

These examples show the importance for the woman to find a person or a group she feels she can trust and talk with and who will provide her with realistic information and give her the opportunity to discuss the ways in which she thinks she may best be helped.

Psychological health

Thirty per cent of the women we talked to, in our survey, who had not reached the menopause were apprehensive or anxious about it, while most of the women who had reached the menopause felt that it was 'better' than they had anticipated. Only 10 per cent of the women considered that the menopausal symptoms were sufficiently distressing to affect severely their day-to-day living.

Many of the women welcomed the menopause as providing relief from distressing premenstrual symptoms, from a chance pregnancy and from menstruation.

Only a few of the women surveyed found the idea of the menopause as unpleasant, and as 'the end of real life'. These women had chosen to see their main role in life as producing, rearing and caring for children. The menopause signalled that this role had largely ceased. The feeling of ceasing to have a significant role after the menopause was increased if the woman's relationship with her partner was unrewarding, and if the woman had few friends and outside interests. It should be stressed that only a very few women had these perceptions.

To many women the menopause also signals that they are getting older. According to women's magazines, getting old is of concern to women as they enter their fourth and fifth decade and particularly their sixth decade. The start of the sixth decade often coincides with menopausal symptoms, and is seen as the major marker of ageing. The menopause does not mean that the woman is old, and that she should now think and behave as an older woman. This was a normal attitude a hundred years ago. It has now largely disappeared, but it persists in some women's minds. If a woman feels that her future stretches out greyly, that she has not done or achieved many of the things she wanted and that her useful life is finished, it often helps if she can talk with other women who have experienced the same problems. Menopause does not signal the end of an active, interesting life or the end of curiosity. It does mark entry into middle age.

Middle age can be a distressing time for some women. A middle-aged woman may realize that she is not as attractive physically as she was when younger; nor is she as physically able to compete with younger women. She may be aware that her relationship with her husband or partner is less than good. The couple may have gone their own ways; they may feel that they have little in common; they no longer talk *with* each other. The woman may no longer even like the man and may wonder how she is going to continue to live with him for the next thirty years or so without a common interest, such as children. She may also wonder how she could manage if she no longer had the financial security he provides. If the woman has no partner the financial problems of middle age may also be present. A single woman may be concerned how to put aside money for retirement or if she is 'made redundant'. She may be concerned about her health, or about the health of a parent for whom she feels responsible.

Children may also be a cause for concern. When a woman reaches the menopausal years, her children are likely to be in their early or mid-twenties, with all the problems that that age can occasion. They may still be involved in risk-taking, of not being responsible, and of being miserable. Whatever advice the woman gives may be seen as wrong, or as interfering, or as not understanding.

Although problems of middle age may occur before, during or after the menopause, many of them can be dealt with by a positive approach.

A positive approach to the menopause

A woman in the menopausal years is experienced and mature. She has coped with many problems, she has solved many problems, and she can be confident that she can cope in the future. The menopausal years are a period when a woman should consider if it is not time that she stopped playing the self-sacrificing role of always considering her needs last. It is often helpful for a woman to make a list of what she has done for others so far in her life, and what she has done for herself. She may get a considerable surprise! It is a period when a woman should make time to decide what makes her feel good, what is comfortable and what she could do to help herself, both psychologically and physically. It is a period when she should take time to reflect on her priorities. For example, most younger women would list their priorities as baby, toddler, children, husband, housework, job, family life and social life. At the end of the list she puts herself and her needs. Middle age, with the menopause as the trigger, can be a time to reassess her priorities and to make changes. Sometimes it is helpful to make a list of the things the woman would like to do and to make enquiries about how to do them. The list may include hobbies, or further education, or exercise programs, or excursions, or sport. Having made her decisions, the woman should ensure that she will do the chosen activity even if she has opposition from her husband or family. The menopausal years are a period when a woman may need to become self assertive and relinquish the role of being someone else's prop.

This is not to suggest that she should antagonize her family. It is a time to talk with her husband, or partner, so that they can make changes, if these are needed to make their relationship more enjoyable. The man may have problems too. He may be concerned about his future career, he may be anxious about his retirement, or his health, he may be concerned about the relationship. The menopausal years give the couple the opportunity to look at their lives, to understand each other's problems, and to reassure each other of their love and concern. The opportunity to be self assertive and to give one's own needs a high priority can be stressful. This and the other stresses of middle age can be reduced by talking to an experienced counsellor and by practising a relaxation technique.

Relaxation exercises

The body benefits from active and from passive forms of relaxation. Active relaxation such as exercise and sport (which is not competitive), walking, jogging, gym workouts, dancing, tennis and swimming are all helpful. A woman who decides on active relaxation should chose an activity she enjoys. If it is strenuous activity (such as gym workouts or jogging) she should have a medical check before starting and should build

up the activity slowly. Some of the active methods of relaxation benefit the cardiovascular system, others do not. Only
those activities that increase the woman's heart rate over a
period of 30 minutes are beneficial in this regard. These
include brisk walking, jogging, and workouts. Tennis, golf and
swimming do not have this effect although they have other
benefits, such as stretching muscles and mobilizing joints.

Passive relaxation is obtained by 'exercises', which may be
done at a community centre or at home. Passive exercises
include yoga, meditation, and hypnosis. One form is becoming
increasingly popular. This is Tai Chi, which consists of passive
relaxation with gentle movements.

A relaxation exercise that is effective in relieving stress and
is easy to do is described below.

Relaxation exercise

1 Sit in a comfortable chair or lie down where you are unlikely to be disturbed for a few minutes.
2 Make sure you are comfortable, with your hands and legs
  uncrossed and with no tight clothing such as shoes or
  belt.
3 Listen to the sounds around you, for example traffic outside, the clock in the room, the family in another room. If
  you are aware of these sounds they will not disturb you
  when you are relaxing.
4 Close your eyes. Although your eyelids may flicker, this
  will stop soon.
5 Become aware of your breathing.
6 Take a breath and then let the rate of your breathing slow,
  so it is about the same as when you are asleep. Don't try to
  force it. Just let it slow down so it is comfortable.
7 Each time you breathe out, let your body relax so you feel
  limp and floppy and warm and heavy as though you are
  sinking into the chair or a bed.
8 Keep thinking about your breathing and keep it slowed
  down.
9 Think of your arm muscles and let them relax. Then think
  of your leg muscles, then your body muscles, then your

neck muscles, your face and forehead muscles — let each group of muscles relax so that you are completely relaxed.

10 Spend no more than 2 minutes doing the exercise, each time you do it.

Try to do this exercise a few times when you do not feel tense. If you find you cannot relax you may wish to join a group that teaches relaxation.

This exercise needs practice — about four to six times a day for a month — so you can use it when you are very tense.

The psychological management of the menopause should take place concurrently with the management of the physical symptoms.

MANAGEMENT OF THE PHYSICAL SYMPTOMS

Women frequently neglect their own health while ensuring that the health of their children and husband or partner is cared for. The presence of a few menopausal symptoms can provide the opportunity for a woman to look at her own health. If a woman has not seen a doctor for some time, and particularly if she feels run down or easily fatigued, the start of the menopausal symptoms is an ideal time to have a health check-up. The woman should choose a doctor in whom she has confidence and who is willing to spend time to answer her questions, no matter how trivial they may seem. The check-up should include an assessment of the woman's weight and blood pressure, and a Pap smear should be taken if this has not been done in the past year. If a woman has not had a mammogram performed, the value of this painless investigation should be discussed. In middle age a person's sight tends to deteriorate, and referral to an ophthalmologist or an optician may be desirable.

Some menopausal women will benefit by improving their nutrition and their eating habits, and this can be talked about at the time of the check-up. We discuss nutrition in Chapter 8. Women of all ages are concerned about their body shape and body weight. A study made in South Australia found that 40 per cent of middle-aged women had been concerned about their weight and had had problems with weight control since their twenties. Over three-quarters of these women wanted to lose weight from parts of their body, most wanting to lose weight from their stomach, their hips or their thighs. This desire can lead to embarking on a variety of diets, or of deciding to eat only 'healthy foods'. In the South Australian study 43 per cent of the women were dieting at the time of the survey.

During the health check-up the woman may seek advice about her intake of caffeine. Caffeine is a component of coffee and of tea, and is found in other drinks such as chocolate, cocoa and cola drinks, in lesser amounts.

Many women are advised to reduce their intake of caffeine in the menopausal years. The advice is because caffeine may increase irritability, lead to insomnia if taken in the 4 to 6 hours before sleeping, and may be a factor in the development of osteoporosis. These effects probably only arise if the woman drinks excessive amounts of caffeine each day (more than eight cups of coffee or tea). Some women find it easy to reduce the quantity, others prefer to change to decaffeinated drinks, others to stop drinking caffeine-containing liquids. Some women feel that they need coffee and drink two cups to 'get started' in the morning. Coffee drinking is also a social event when a woman meets with her friends. If she doesn't join in she may feel uncomfortable and an 'outsider'. The aim should be to reduce the amount of caffeine ingested in a way that doesn't interfere with the woman's life style too much, and not to make the woman feel guilty about drinking any coffee or tea.

In the health check-up the question of smoking tobacco should be raised. Although in the past 10 years fewer adult women are smoking, tobacco-induced lung cancer is increasing among middle-aged women. Unfortunately tobacco is an addictive drug and many people find it difficult to break the habit. A cigarette may be a solace in moments of stress. However, as there is some evidence that in some women hot flushes may be aggravated by cigarette smoking, the menopausal years may be a time when it is easier to break the addiction.

The general health check-up should lead to a discussion with the health professional about the specific symptoms that are affecting the woman. As we noted in Chapter 5, hot flushes and a dry or painful vagina are the only confirmed physical symptoms associated with the menopause. If the hot flush occurs at night, when a woman is in bed, well insulated by bedclothes, the raised body temperature during the flush may cause her to sweat and to wake up. If she does she may find it difficult to go to sleep again. In other words, she develops insomnia. But if the hot flushes are relieved by treatment, the night sweats and the insomnia will also be relieved.

OESTROGEN TREATMENT

Hot flushes and menopausal vaginal symptoms can be treated effectively by taking oestrogen. The oestrogen should be taken in the smallest effective amount to avoid over-stimulation of the uterus and breasts. However, because bone loss is often great during the first 5 to 10 years after the meno-pause, oestrogen should be taken for this period of time. This use of oestrogen for osteoporosis is discussed further in Chapter 9.

Which oestrogen to use?

The pharmacological manufacturers have produced three groups of oestrogen for the treatment of menopausal symptoms. These are (1) synthetic oestrogens; (2) equine oes-trogens and (3) the so-called 'natural' oestrogens (see Table 6.1)

The synthetic oestrogens are produced by a chemical pro-cess from a steroid that has 18 carbon atoms (oestrane). Although they are similar to the body's natural oestrogen (17-beta oestradiol) in their biological action, they are not found in any natural system. The two synthetic oestrogens currently used in treatment of the menopause are ethinyl oestradiol and its derivative, mestranol. The synthetic oestrogens are absorbed rapidly into the body but metabolize (break-down) slowly and with difficulty; they stimulate liver enzymes more than do the oestrogens of the other two groups.

The equine oestrogens (also known as conjugated equine oestrogens) are derived from the urine of mares, and in this

Table 6.1: Oestrogen preparations currently available for the treatment of menopausal symptoms and the prevention of osteoporosis

Preparation	Trade name	Dose per day
Oral preparations		
'Natural' oestrogens:		
Piperazine oestrone sulphate (estropipate)	Ogen, Harmogen	0.625–5.0 mg
Oestradiol valerate	Progynova	1.0–2.0 mg
Oestradiol (micronized)	Estace	1.0–2.0 mg
Oestriol	Ovestrin	1.0–4.0 mg
Equine oestrogens	Premarin	0.3–2.5 mg
Synthetic oestrogens:		
Ethinyl oestradiol	Estigen; Feminone Lynoral; Primogen	0.01–0.03 mg
Transdermal oestrogens	Estraderm	0.05–1.0 mg. The patch is changed every 4 days
Implants	Oestradiol	20 mg every 30 weeks or 50 mg every 52 weeks
Vaginal preparations	Dienoestrol cream Kolpon pessaries Premarin cream	½ applicator daily or less often
Combined preparations		
Oestradiol valerate and levonorgestrel	Cycloprogynova	one tablet daily
Conjugated equine oestrogen and norgestrel	Prempak	,,
Oestradiol (micronized) and norethisterone acetate	Kliogest	,,
Oestrogen and testosterone		
Ethinyl oestradiol and methyltestosterone	Mixogen	1–2 tablets daily for 21 days; 7 days no drug; repeat.

sense they are natural. The principal hormone in equine oestrogens is equilin, which is not made by humans and has no biological effect in a woman's body, but there is sufficient amount of oestradiol in the substance to make conjugated equine oestrogens a useful product.

The so-called natural oestrogens, although made in the laboratory, are called 'natural' because their metabolism is very similar to that of oestrogens produced by the body.

With several oestrogen preparations available (Table 6.1), a woman and her doctor might reasonably ask: 'Which oestrogen preparation is the safest and the most effective?' The drug manufacturers naturally want doctors to believe that their product is superior to any of the others available, that it is the safest and that it produces the fewest undesirable side-effects. Drug manufacturers research their new drugs in a responsible way and the research is controlled by government institutions, to make sure that the new drug is as safe as it is humanly possible to be.

In studying the effects on the body of oestrogen preparations, the pharmaceutical manufacturers have looked at very many biochemical and metabolic changes that occur in a woman's body. In collaboration with doctors, they have investigated the prevalence of the undesirable side-effects in their product. This research is of immense value and importance but the results are often interpreted by the sales division of the pharmaceutical company in ways that are rather devious. This is understandable, as the manufacturers invest a large amount of money in developing a new product to the stage at which it is available to treat a condition. Unless they can recoup their investment they are likely to go out of business.

If the voluminous medical literature regarding the available oestrogen preparations is scrutinized carefully and critically, there is surprisingly little difference between the biochemical and metabolic effects of the various preparations, provided the dose of each oestrogen is equivalent (equipotent) (Table 6.2). There is also surprisingly little difference between their undesirable side-effects.

A possible exception to this is that ethinyl oestradiol is broken down (metabolized) in the body more slowly than the so-called 'natural' oestrogens, so that its effect lasts longer.

Table 6.2: Equivalent doses of various oestrogen preparations, taken by mouth, to relieve menopausal symptoms

Ethinyl oestradiol	0.01 mg (10μg)
Conjugated equine oestrogens	0.625 mg
Piperazine oestrone sulphate	1.5 mg
Oestradiol valerate	2.0 mg
Oestriol hemisuccinate	4.0 mg

Because of this, ethinyl oestradiol (and to a lesser extent conjugated equine oestrogens) may alter certain liver enzymes and perhaps liver function. In contrast, the 'natural' oestrogens have only a small effect on liver function. But whether or not these changes of liver function are important clinically is not clear.

Some doctors believe that an alteration in liver function predisposes to high blood pressure, to gall bladder disease, to high blood lipid levels and to an increased ability of the blood to clot. This may cause a clot to form in a vein (thrombosis). More rarely, a clot may detach and reach the lungs, causing a pulmonary embolus. Other doctors believe that the alteration in liver function is an interesting observation but has little clinical significance. They point out that if the changes are dangerous to a woman, the 50 million women taking the contraceptive pill are at risk. This is because the oestrogen used in the pill is ethinyl oestradiol and the dose taken for 21 days every month is higher than that taken each month by menopausal women.

The arguments against this belief are that women taking the pill are younger, so the risk of thrombosis in veins is less, and that the pill contains progestogen (a synthetic form of the hormone, progesterone), which may counteract the effects of oestrogen on blood clotting. However, this argument is invalid as menopausal women are also prescribed a progestogen, which is usually taken for 10 to 14 days each month.

At present there is no evidence that any one formulation of oestrogen is better than any other in eliminating menopausal symptoms, and it doesn't matter much which one is prescribed. The doctor's preference, the woman's wishes and the cost of the formulation should be assessed, before choosing the oestrogen preparation favoured.

How oestrogens are prescribed

Most doctors prescribe oestrogen tablets or capsules, which the woman takes by mouth. A few doctors give oestrogen tablets that are absorbed from the vagina, and a few 'implant' oestrogen tablets under the skin. Recently a new oestrogen preparation has been developed that is absorbed from a 'patch' fixed to the skin.

An advantage of the last three ways of prescribing oestrogen over oestrogens taken by mouth is that oral oestrogens are absorbed from the gut and are first carried to the liver. As has been mentioned, they may induce the production of liver proteins and enzymes. As well, a variable portion of the oestrogen is inactivated in the liver and consequently produces no beneficial effect. The inactivity may be overcome by giving a larger dose of oestrogen or by changing the chemical nature of the oestrogen so that less is inactivated. One way of achieving this is to make the oestrogen particles very small, by 'micronizing' them. This is a process in which the substances are broken down into tiny particles, which are absorbed into the body more easily and are less likely to be inactivated before they have had their effect. Micronized oestrogen can be taken by mouth or placed in the vagina.

Vaginal oestrogen Oestrogen tablets or creams placed in the vagina are readily absorbed into the body. An example of this absorption has been reported from Sweden. The scientists found that 0.2 mg of the micronized oestradiol placed in the vagina produced the blood levels of oestrogen found in a woman during the first half of her menstrual cycle. If the micronized oestradiol was given by mouth, ten times the dose was needed to produce the same result.

This means that if oestrogen is given vaginally, the dose must be reduced. Many menopausal women do not like placing tablets or cream in their vagina, so that the vaginal route is usually only chosen if the woman's main complaint is vaginal dryness, burning or discomfort. Of course, the hormone is equally effective for these symptoms if given by one of the other routes, provided the dose is adjusted.

Transdermal systems of giving oestrogen This is a new

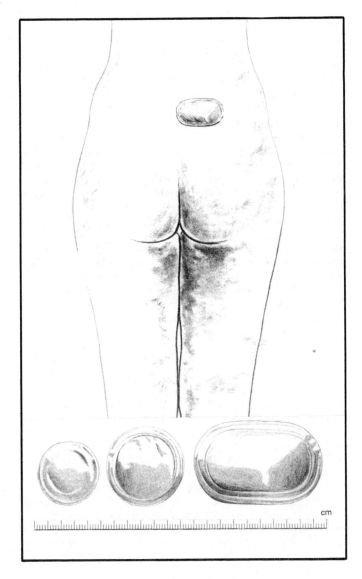

Figure 6.1: Transdermal oestrogen

development which has several advantages. Oestradiol (in a 0.05 or 0.1mg dose) is mixed in a solvent gel and is applied to the skin in a 'plastic' patch, which sticks to the skin (Fig. 6.1). The oestrogen is absorbed through the skin and enters the blood circulation. Oestrogen patches are stuck to the skin on the woman's abdomen or between her buttocks, and are peeled off and replaced every 3 or 4 days. Apart from slight redness under the patch, experienced by a few women (rather like that some women get under a Band-aid), no problems have been reported.

The lower dose of oestrogen is chosen first. The woman keeps a record of the number of hot flushes she experiences each day. If the number has not fallen to less than two a day in 2 weeks, the dose of oestrogen is doubled.

Oestrogen injections and 'implants' A few women prefer to have an injection of a 'long acting oestrogen' every 3 to 4 weeks. 'Pellets' of oestrogen, which are implanted under the skin about every 6 months (Fig. 6.2), are also available. These preparations release a small quantity of oestrogen into the woman's circulation each day so that the she does not have to remember to take a daily tablet or to place a 'patch' on her skin every 3 or 4 days.

There is a problem about this method. The level of oestrogen in the blood varies greatly in different women who have an oestrogen implant. As the aim is to keep the blood level in the range found before menopause, the variability can cause problems. Some women may have too high levels (which are potentially dangerous); other women may have too low levels, so they have inadequate protection against osteoporosis, for example. This suggests that women who chose to have an oestrogen implant should have a blood test every 3 months, to check if a new implant is needed.

A few doctors add the male hormone, testosterone, to the oestrogen implant claiming that the testosterone improves the muscle tone of postmenopausal women and increases their sexual desire and responsiveness. Considerable doubt exists whether testosterone is responsible for an increase in libido (see Chapter 13).

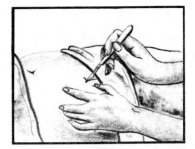

Under a local anaesthetic a small incision is made through
the skin of the abdomen

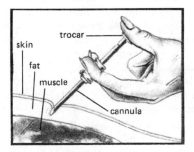

A trocar and cannula are pushed through the incision into
the tissue between the skin and the muscle; the trocar is then
withdrawn

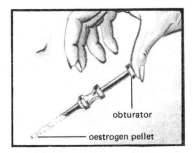

The hormone pellet is injected into the tissue through the
cannula

Figure 6.2: Oestrogen implant

PROGESTOGENS

During the reproductive years of a woman's life, following ovulation the hormone progesterone is produced. Progesterone reduces the stimulating (and perhaps cancer-producing) effects of unopposed oestrogen on the tissues of the genital tract and the breasts.

Synthetic progesterone-like substances — called progestogens — are equally effective in protecting a woman's tissues against the undesirable effects of oestrogen. They have the advantage that they can be given by mouth, while 'natural progesterone' must be given by injection or absorbed from the vagina, although recently a preparation of progesterone that is effective by mouth has been developed.

To protect menopausal women from the undesirable effects of administered oestrogen, a progestogen should be taken for at least 12 to 14 days each month.

Several types of progestogen are available currently (Table 6.3). Proponents of each claim that their particular progestogen is superior, but in reality there is little difference. In the USA, medroxyprogesterone acetate is preferred, as the product is thought to alter blood lipids less than the others. However, a Swedish study suggests that the difference found is due to the use of a larger than necessary daily dose of norethisterone or levonorgestrel. Some doctors prefer to use one of these two products, as medroxyprogesterone acetate (in the recommended daily dose of 5–10 mg) is less effective in suppressing the oestrogen-induced changes in endometrial cells. New progestogens that have no effect on blood lipids are becoming available (desorgestrel, gestodene and norgestimate). These may replace the older progestogens in the near future.

The administration of a progestogen for 12 to 14 days each month may cause problems in a few women. In these women the progestogen produces negative feelings of irritability, fatigue or depression while oestrogen induces positive feelings of well being. The matter is complex, because women treated with large doses of progestogen for cancer do not report the negative feelings. If the findings are confirmed it is clear that the dose of progestogen should be the lowest

Table 6.3: Progestogens currently available for hormone treatment in the menopausal years

Name	Trade name	Dose (mg a day) (taken for 14 days each month)
Norethisterone	Primolut N	1.0*–2.5 mg
	Micronor	0.35*–0.70 mg
Medroxyprogesterone acetate	Provera	10 mg
Levonorgestrel	Microlut Microval }	0.7*–1.25 mg
Desorgestrel	Gestrinone	0.125 mg
Micronized progesterone (in capsules)	Uterogestan	200 mg

* Dose that is usually sufficient to supress oestrogen effect on the uterus and endometrium.

needed to prevent the undesirable 'stimulating' effect of oestrogen on the tissues of the breast and the uterus.

A problem associated with the use of a progestogen is that one woman in five develops some degree of abdominal bloating, and two in three have a monthly bleed!

Experiments are continuing to find ways of avoiding these side effects.

HORMONE REPLACEMENT TREATMENT

It is clear from the above that whichever route of oestrogen is chosen by the woman, after discussion with her doctor, she should take one of the progestogen preparations (or micronized progesterone if she wishes) for 12 to 14 days each month to prevent the possible development of uterine (endometrial) cancer.

Together, oestrogen and progestogen supplements are often called hormone replacement treatment.

The regimens of hormone replacement treatment

Most doctors in the USA prescribe oestrogen for 21 days each month and add a progestogen for the last 12 days. The patient takes no hormones for 7 days (during which she may have a recurrence of her symptoms and, usually, a 'withdrawal' bleed).

This regimen is also followed by some doctors in Australia and Europe, although recently increasing numbers of doctors are recommending that the woman takes the oestrogen each day without a break, and takes the progestogen for the first 14 days each month. During this time, preferably after the 11th day of the month, the woman may expect to have a withdrawal bleed. If bleeding occurs in the first 10 days of progestogen treatment, the dose should be increased.

A group of Dutch gynaecologists have carried this process further. They prescribe oestrogen to be taken daily and only add a progestogen for 14 days every 3 months. They claim that this reduces the side effects of progestogen treatment (abdominal bloating and 'periods'), without reducing the protection progestogen gives to the tissues. This must be considered experimental until further evidence of the safety of the regimen is obtained.

A few doctors prescribe oestrogen and progestogen, which their patients take daily. .

Effectiveness of hormone replacement treatment

The most obvious way to judge the effectiveness of oestrogen treatment is that the hot flushes or the burning feeling in the vagina cease or are much reduced. However, a way of determining the effectiveness of treatment was (and is) used by many doctors, particularly in Europe and the USA, who claim it is more 'scientific'. The method is to calculate the 'maturity index' of the vaginal epithelium. The thickness of the vaginal wall can be deduced from the type of vaginal cells shed into the vaginal cavity. The proponents of this method believe the appearance and number of the various cells show the degree of oestrogen circulating in the woman's body. It is true that development or maturation of the vaginal epithelium depends on the level of circulating oestrogen, but once a quantum of oestrogen is circulating, the relationship ceases.

Despite this, many doctors believe that a vaginal swab should be taken from all menopausal women to help plan

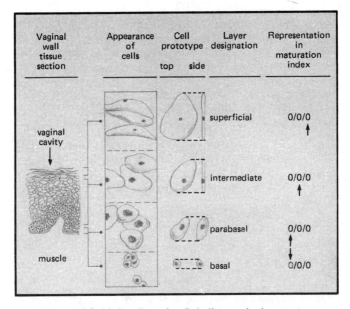

Figure 6.3: Maturation of cells in the vaginal mucosa

treatment and at intervals when the woman is receiving oestrogen to check the effectiveness of treatment. The swab is
smeared onto a slide, stained and examined through a microscope. The slide shows the types of cells that make up the
vaginal wall in differing proportions (Fig. 6.3).

By counting the proportion of each cell type in the smear, a
'maturation index' is obtained. The higher the proportion of
parabasal cells, the greater the need for treatment; the higher
the proportion of superficial cells, the greater the effect of
oestrogen. Recent studies have shown that this test is of little
or no value in determining the dose required or the duration of
oestrogen treatment. It has no place in the management of the
menopause.

Investigations needed before taking hormone replacement treatment

As in any medical procedure, the doctor should take a history enquiring about general health, high blood pressure, diabetes, smoking habits, exercise and so on. A physical examination, including a vaginal examination is essential.

Until recently, many menopausal women had their uterus curetted under an anaesthetic to remove the entire endometrial lining. Alternatively, a specimen of the uterine lining was taken without an anaesthetic. This procedure is called an endometrial biopsy, and involves the insertion of a small tube into the uterus to extract a piece of the endometrium, which can then be examined microscopically to make sure that there is no abnormality in the cells. Recent experience has shown that if the woman is given oestrogen, and progestogen for at least 12 days each month, the procedure is not required nor justified.

A few American physicians give a small dose of a progestogen (medroxyprogesterone acetate 10 mg) for 5 days before starting oestrogen treatment. If no bleeding occurs within 7 days of the progestogen, treatment is started. However, if bleeding occurs, an endometrial biopsy is made, although cancer is rarely found (1 in 1000 times).

Most women can safely be prescribed oestrogen treatment after checking that (1) the breasts have no lumps; (2) the blood pressure is normal; (3) there is no enlargement of the internal genital organs; (4) there is no history of irregular bleeding from the uterus.

Certain women should not be prescribed oestrogen for the reasons listed in Table 6.4

Principles regarding hormone replacement treatment

There is no doubt that oestrogens will relieve a woman's menopausal symptoms dramatically. This statement applies particularly to the 'cascade' of hot flushes → night sweats → insomnia, and to the vaginal symptoms. Some studies claim that oestrogens improve the mental ability of a menopausal woman (see Chapter 12). Oestrogens are also of great benefit in preventing bone loss in the decade after the menopause, thus preventing osteoporosis (see Chapter 9).

So that the undesirable side-effects of oestrogen are mini-

Table 6.4: Contra-indications to oestrogen treatment

Women who have or have had the following illnesses should not be prescribed oestrogen:
* Acute liver disease
* Chronic liver disease with impaired function
* Breast cancer
* A history of two or more episodes of acute deep venous thrombosis

Women who have or have had the following illnesses may take oestrogen but require frequent checks:
* High blood pressure
* Benign breast disease
* Uterine 'fibroids'
* Migraine
* Gall bladder disease
* Chronic thrombophlebitis
* Endometriosis
* Familial high blood lipids

mized, the following principles should be understood by the woman and her doctor:

● Oestrogen should be taken in the lowest effective dose
● Progestogens should be taken with oestrogen at periodic intervals (currently 12 to 14 days each month) to protect the woman against possible uterine (endometrial) cancer and possible breast cancer
● with this treatment, over 60 per cent of menopausal women will have monthly 'periods' — these are usually scanty and last about 3 days
● provided the bleeds are regular, no concern need be expressed, but if the bleeding becomes irregular in duration or onset, it is likely that the woman's doctor will recommend a curettage
● In general, the combination of oestrogen with other hormones or drugs is unnecessary — the exception being a progestogen. There is no evidence that the addition of testosterone is of any benefit.

Adherence by the woman, on the advice of her doctor, to these guidelines, makes oestrogen treatment an appropriate and effective method of controlling hot flushes. She is asked to record how many times a day the hot flushes occur, and if the frequency has not fallen to below five after 7 days of treatment, she doubles the dose, taking two tablets each day instead of one. The dose may need to be increased a further step before control is obtained. Some of the pharmaceutical manufacturers are aware of this and provide tablets of different strengths.

The correct dose of progestogen is also important. Too little is ineffective; too much increases the chance of side effects.

The available progestogens are shown in Table 6.3 on page 51. To avoid side-effects, the lowest dose should be given initially. If this leads to a bleed each month on or after the 11th day of taking the progestogen the dose is adequate. If bleeding occurs before day 11, the dose is insufficient to make sure that the endometrium is not being unduly stimulated and the dose should be doubled.

Other possible treatments

Is there any treatment for hot flushes in women who cannot take oestrogens?

Two other forms of treatment for hot flushes are available, although neither is as effective as oestrogen in relieving the symptoms. The first is to use a drug normally prescribed to reduce high blood pressure. The drug is called clonidine (Dixarit). Clonidine reduces the responsiveness of blood vessels, so that they dilate less readily. As vasodilatation precedes a hot flush, its control reduces the frequency of the symptom. Clonidine is more effective if given in the form of a skin patch (transdermal system).

The second treatment is for the woman to take one of the progestogen drugs, either norethisterone (5 mg daily) or medroxyprogesterone (Provera) 10 to 20 mg daily. Either of these hormones seems to reduce the frequency of hot flushes, by half to three-quarters, but does not eliminate them as effectively as oestrogen.

APPENDIX

Oestrogen metabolism

Some readers may wish to know more about the way in which the oestrogens are metabolized in the body; this appendix will help them to understand the processes.

In the body, three main oestrogens circulate. They are: *oestradiol*, which is the most active form; *oestrone*, which is less active; and *oestriol*, which is a relatively very weak oestrogen.

Oestradiol is synthesized in the ovaries and enters the blood bound to a carrier protein. It is carried to certain 'target' cells, which have 'receptors' and bind onto the oestrogen. It is then absorbed into the target cells.

In the target cell, oestradiol is converted into oestrone, a less active oestrogen, which is transferred to the nucleus of the cell where it alters the cell's processes through a complicated series of changes.

Oestrone is kept in store in the body as oestrone sulphate, and is also the form in which oestrogens are excreted from the body. There are several chemical pathways by which oestrone is metabolized. A major pathway converts oestrone into oestriol. This oestrogen was thought to be relatively inactive biologically, but it is now known that if it is given over a period of time it has biological effects similar to those of oestradiol and oestrone.

Two other metabolic pathways are also biologically important. In the first, oestrone is converted into 2-hydroxyoestrone. This substance is a catecholoestrogen and is probably the biological form in which oestrogen is taken up by, and is active in, the brain. It is also the major breakdown product of oestradiol found in the urine. In the second of these pathways oestrone is metabolized into 4-hydroxyoestrone. This substance binds easily to oestrogen receptors in tissues (although not as easily as oestradiol and 2-hydroxyoestrone), but its biological actions have not yet been clarified.

EFFECTS OF OESTROGENS ON THE LIVER

The several types of oestrogens available to treat the menopause (see Table 6.1) may be given by mouth, by injection, absorbed from the vagina or given through the skin. If they are given by mouth, the oestrogen is absorbed from the gut and carried to the liver, as over 90 per cent of blood that has supplied the gut passes through the liver. If oestrogens are given by injection, absorbed through the vagina or given through the skin, the effects on the liver are minimized, as only 10 per cent of the blood passes through the liver. By avoiding having to pass through the liver, the ratio of oestradiol to oestrone in the blood becomes much more like the ratio that occurs in a woman's body in the years before the menopause. However, as mentioned, oestrone sulphate, and conjugated equine oestrogen have to pass through the liver before they become biologically active, so there is no benefit in giving either of these drugs except by mouth.

Each type of synthetic oestrogen affects liver function in a different way.

Ethinyl oestradiol   This oestrogen is readily absorbed from the gut when taken by mouth, and is carried to the liver. The liver cells preferentially take up twice the amount of ethinyl oestradiol compared with that taken up by the uterus. This means that the amount of ethinyl oestradiol in the liver will be at least twice that in any other organ irrespective of its route of administration. Ethinyl oestradiol is also metabolized slowly so that its effect on liver function is greater than that of the other synthetic oestrogens.

'Natural' oestrogens   The effect of the so-called 'natural' oestrogens on liver function depends on the route of administration and on the type of oestrogen. *Piperazine oestrone sulphate*, for example, is only effective when taken by mouth, because the piperazine portion blocks the biological function of the oestrone until it is removed. Piperazine is added to enhance absorption of the compound from the gut and is removed in the liver. After its removal, oestrone sulphate, which is also an inert oestrogen, remains. Liver enzymes remove the sulphate leaving the active oestrone.

Conjugated equine oestrogen   This is obtained from the urine of pregnant mares. It is a mixture of oestrogens — 65 per cent being oestrone sulphate and 35 per cent is equilin, an oestrogen not found in humans. As with piperazine oestrone sulphate, it has to pass through the liver to have the sulphate removed and become biologically active. In the liver, conjugated equine oestrogens induce liver protein production, to a greater extent than do the so-called 'natural' oestrogens, but less than does ethinyl oestradiol. Premarin has been called a natural oestrogen, but it is not. It is a natural oestrogen in horses, not humans!

Oestradiol valerate   This compound is absorbed readily because of the valerate which, on reaching the liver, is removed, leaving active oestradiol.

Micronized oestradiol   This form of oestradiol is readily absorbed because of the 'micro' size of its particles. It then passes through the liver on its way to target cells without being further altered.

Oestriol   Oestriol is also available to treat menopausal symptoms, It is a very weak oestrogen and large doses are needed.

7

THE SIDE-EFFECTS OF HORMONAL TREATMENT

Oestrogens are hormones; they enter cells that have special areas on their surface (receptors) enabling the hormone to 'bind' to the cell. The cells that have the largest number of receptors for oestrogen are those of the genital tract and the breast milk-ducts. Inside the cells, oestrogen is transferred to the nucleus of the cell where it stimulates cell growth. In this way oestrogen may interfere with the normal life of the cell and may possibly promote cancer in tissues that have many oestrogen receptors, such as the lining of the uterus and the glandular tissues of the breasts.

Oestrogen is secreted by the ovaries throughout a woman's fertile years, that is from about 13 to 50 years of age, but endometrial cancer and breast cancer are uncommon during these years. The reason that cancer is unusual is because the second female sex hormone, progesterone, which is also secreted by the ovary, controls and counteracts the stimulating effect of oestrogen.

CANCER OF THE ENDOMETRIUM

The possible cancer-producing effect of oestrogen was not recognized in the 1960s and 1970s, when many menopausal women were prescribed oestrogen tablets to help them remain 'forever feminine'. Then in 1975, three reports produced evidence that oestrogen taken in this way, without taking a progestogen as well to 'oppose' the oestrogen led to endometrial cancer in a number of women. A woman taking oestrogen daily for 3 or 4 years had three times the chance of developing endometrial cancer compared with a woman not taking oestrogen. The actual risk increased from 1 per 1000 women to 3 per 1000 women. These findings were disputed by many doctors at the time and a controversy followed. But they have been shown to be correct. Since 1975, seventeen carefully conducted studies have been made, all but one of which have confirmed that unopposed oestrogen treatment is associated with an increased risk that the woman will develop endometrial cancer, but if she does, the cancer is usually curable by surgery.

The results of these investigations and the concern that oestrogen treatment might be dangerous has led to a change in the hormonal treatment of the menopause. It is now current medical practice for menopausal women who have the symptoms of hot flushes (and the 'cascade' symptoms of night sweats and insomnia) or a painful vagina and who are taking oestrogen, to take, in addition, a small dose of progestogen for 12 to 14 days each month. This regimen effectively prevents oestrogen stimulating the endometrial cells unduly. The woman has no increased risk of developing endometrial cancer compared with women of a similar age who do not take oestrogens.

There is a problem. Over 90 per cent of women who take the oestrogen–progestogen combination will have a 'withdrawal' bleed (usually scanty and lasting 3–4 days) during the treatment-free week, or during the time they are taking the progestogen. These 'periods' may annoy some women who had hoped that their menstrual periods would cease with the menopause. The advantage of having a withdrawal bleed is that it is a useful sign that the endometrium is not being stimulated excessively by oestrogen. If the bleed occurs before the 11th day of the oestrogen–progestogen combination, the dose of progestogen needs to be increased. If it occurs on or after the 11th day, it indicates that the risk of endometrial cancer developing is negligible.

Some doctors believe, as an added precaution to make sure that cancer does not develop, that any woman receiving oestrogen treatment should have a sample of the endometrium (a biopsy) taken every year. This can be done without an anaesthetic by introducing a narrow metal tube into the uterus and extracting a piece of the endometrium. Most women who have had the procedure done say the discomfort is slight, but about 20 per cent of women find it painful and 15 per cent find it very painful. The degree of pain and discomfort is reduced if the woman is given a capsule of mefenamic acid (Ponstan) half an hour before the procedure is made. An alternative is to admit the woman to hospital and curette her uterus under a general anaesthetic. This is costly, invasive, and time-consuming.

Doctors who do not recommend an annual endometrial biopsy have several reasons for this. First, less than one woman in every 1000 in this age group develops endometrial cancer. Based on routine sampling of menopausal women, it was found that over half of those women in whom cancer was diagnosed had symptoms. In other words, they had irregular bleeding before curettage. This means that to detect one endometrial cancer in those women who have no symptoms, over 2000 endometrial curettes would have to be made. Second, as progestogen is now given routinely, the possible cancer-producing effect of oestrogen is inhibited. Thus *routine* endometrial curettage is not required, but if a woman taking oestrogen treatment develops irregular, unscheduled bleeding, endometrial curettage is essential.

BREAST CANCER

The question whether oestrogen treatment increases a woman's chance of developing breast cancer is very important because the growth of many forms of breast cancer seem to be increased by oestrogen, and breast cancer is one of the more common cancers in older women. The main problem in answering the question has been to devise a methodologically sound study. This has proved difficult. At present the consensus of opinion is that oestrogen used to treat menopausal symptoms are unlikely to cause breast cancer, even if the woman takes the oestrogen for a long period of time, but as a precaution progestogen should be taken for 10 to 14 days each month. This means that women can safely take oestrogen together with progestogen, but should examine their breasts each month, have an annual breast check from a doctor and a mammogram each year.

CARDIOVASCULAR DISEASE

Four times as many men as women under the age of 50 die from heart attacks. This suggests that in some way oestrogens protect women from cardiovascular disease. Against this was the observation that after the age of 35, oestrogens may increase the likelihood of a woman developing a blood clot in a vein and possibly a pulmonary embolus. The effect of oestrogen on the incidence of heart disease and on that of deep venous thrombosis is difficult to study because many other factors are involved.

Thrombosis

Several studies have shown that the risk of venous thrombosis and pulmonary embolism is increased among women taking oestrogen-containing compounds. However, the dose of oestrogen given was much larger than that commonly required to control menopausal symptoms. Among menopausal women taking oestrogens or oestrogen–progestogen combinations, most investigators have found no alteration in the blood factors that lead to blood clotting, whichever oestrogen preparation is prescribed, provided the dose was equivalent (equipotent). Clinical experience in the use of oestrogens to treat menopausal symptoms for long periods of time indicates that such treatment is not associated with an increase in deep vein thrombosis.

HIGH BLOOD PRESSURE

In a small number of women, hormone replacement treatment provokes a rise in blood pressure, so that the woman develops hypertension. If the woman stops treatment, the blood pressure falls to within the normal range. The chance of developing hypertension is one of the reasons why a menopausal woman should see her doctor every year, so that her blood pressure, her breasts and her cervix may be checked.

GALL BLADDER DISEASE

The incidence of gall bladder disease is increased slightly among women who take oestrogen for long periods to relieve menopausal symptoms. The increase is small and other factors such as obesity and diet are more significant.

8

A HEALTHY DIET FOR THE MENOPAUSE AND AFTER

As people grow older there is a tendency for them to put on weight, women being more affected than men. Studies in the USA show that an average white woman gains 10 kg between the ages of 15 and 50. By the age of the menopause, about 30 per cent of women are overweight and about 9 per cent are obese. Obesity carries certain health hazards, such as an increased chance of developing mature-onset diabetes; an increased chance of developing gall bladder disease; a greater likelihood of developing high blood pressure, and a greater chance of having a heart attack or a stroke. Obesity also means that if a woman develops arthritis, the strain on the affected joint is increased and the disability is greater.

Women are prone to put on weight in middle age for two main reasons. First, they are likely to be less active than when younger. Second, they are more likely than men to indulge in sweetened drinks (including coffee and tea) and to eat energy-rich snacks between meals.

The contribution of a balanced diet to health is being increasingly recognized, and each year an expert committee in some developed country issues a report suggesting the most appropriate mix of food that should be eaten for health. Unfortunately, the advice is often too obscure to be followed, or makes eating too unpalatable, so the recommendations are largely ignored by people in the community.

DIETARY PRINCIPLES

It is important for a woman passing through the menopause, as in other periods of her life, to eat a healthy diet. It is known that only 10 per cent of obese people who decide to diet are able to reduce their weight by more than 10 kg (22 lbs) , and fewer are able to maintain the lower weight for a year or longer. The reason is that many diets are dull, or 'faddish', or inappropriate. For this reason, rather than prescribe a diet, the principles of a healthy, balanced diet will be given in this chapter, and the reader may then choose whether or not to follow these principles.

If you want to eat a healthy diet (see Fig 8.1), you should try to follow these recommendations:

- Limit the amount of fat in your diet by choosing lean meat, usually by grilling food rather than frying it, and by limiting the quantity of cakes and biscuits that you eat.
- Reduce the amount of sugar you eat, including sugar 'hidden' in cakes, confectionery and soft drinks.
- Eat more 'complex' carbohydrates, that is eat more whole-grain bread, more oatmeal, more vegetables and more fruit. This increases the amount of fibre in your diet (and is preferable to adding wheat bran to your diet).
- Use less salt by reducing the amount used in cooking and by trying not to add salt to the food on your plate.
- Increase your intake of calcium.

Reducing dietary fat

In Australia and Britain, about 38 per cent of the total energy eaten comes from fat. Nutritionists recommend that the percentage should be reduced to 34 per cent. Fat carries twice as much energy as carbohydrates and this is stored in the body, so that the person may become obese. Also, fats, particularly saturated fats, are implicated in the development of heart disease, which becomes more likely to occur as women become postmenopausal. Fat is eaten when you choose fatty meat, and particularly when you eat fried foods. Fat is also 'hidden' in cakes, shortenings, ice-cream, pastries and biscuits (cookies), and chocolates.

You can reduce the amount of fat you eat, and particularly

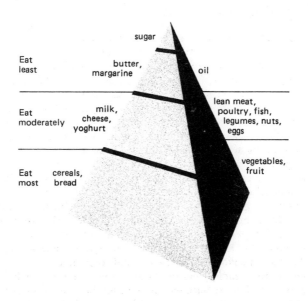

sugar

Eat
least

butter,
margarine

oil

lean meat,
poultry, fish,
legumes, nuts,
eggs

Eat
moderately

milk,
cheese,
yoghurt

vegetables,
fruit

Eat
most

cereals,
bread

Figure 8.1: Healthy diet pyramid

the amount of the more dangerous saturated fats, relatively easily. And it need not disturb your usual eating habits too much. To do this, you may choose lean beef and mutton and try to avoid processed meats like sausages, which have a high proportion of saturated fat. You should eat more fish and poultry and try to resist the temptation to eat the skin because it is fatty.

Usually when you cook meat, poultry or fish it should be grilled or casseroled rather than fried. It is better to use sunflower seed oil or safflower seed oil rather than lard, beef dripping or olive oil. Lard and dripping have a lot of saturated fat in them and olive oil has a fair amount.

It is preferable to choose polyunsaturated margarine (make sure the margarine you buy is polyunsaturated) rather than butter. But if you enjoy butter you may eat it if you spread it thinly.

It will also help if you eat fewer cakes and less confectionery, as these foods are 'energy rich' and contain hidden fat and hidden sugar.

Reducing sugar in the diet

Sugar and other 'refined carbohydrates' (that is cereal from which most of the fibre has been removed) are a readily available source of energy, the excess of which is stored as fat and adds to the risk that you will become obese. You can reduce the amount of sugar you eat if you do the following:

- Start by cutting down the number of spoons of sugar you add to your tea or coffee, and over a few weeks cut out all sugar you add to hot drinks. What you are doing is 'desensitizing' your taste buds' demands for a sweet taste. This is also a problem if you choose a sugar substitute. It provides no energy but it does not stop your taste buds demanding a sweet taste.
- If you eat breakfast cereals don't put sugar on them.
- Avoid eating cakes and sweet biscuits, except on special occasions.
- Cut out ordinary soft drinks, drink low-calorie ones instead. They do contain sweeteners, but the amount of cyclamate or saccharin in them is not going to do you any harm.
- Or better, buy citrus fruit and make your own fruit drink instead. The fructose in the fruit will make it sweet enough and you will not need to add additional sucrose.
- If you drink alcohol, choose the lighter (less sugary) varieties of beer and avoid ginger-ale, bitter lemon and tonic in your brandy or gin. The first is very sweet; the others seem to be bitter but in reality are loaded with hidden sugar.
- Stop eating sweets, chocolates and toffees between meals. If you need to chew something, chew an apple.

But don't be obsessive. If you want to eat a cake or a piece of chocolate or some ice-cream or have a soft drink from time to time — you can!

The need for fibre in the diet

For a long time, fibre, that is the outer part of many cereals, vegetables and fruits, was considered to be of no nutritional value. Now it is known that the lack of fibre in modern Western

Table 8.1: Best sources of dietary fibre

	Average serving size	Dietary fibre (g)
Bread and cereals:		
All-bran	30 g (1 oz)	7.5
Muesli	60 g (2 oz)	4.0
Raw bran	7 g (2½ level tablespoons)	3.0
Oatmeal	30 g (1 oz) raw	2.0
Wholemeal bread	30 g (1 oz; 1 slice)	2.5
White bread	30 g (1 oz; 1 slice)	1.0
Wholemeal pasta	60 g (2 oz) dry weight	5.5
Fruit:		
Orange	180 g (6 oz; 1 piece)	3.6
Banana	180 g (6 oz; 1 piece)	3.5
Apple	150 g (5 oz; 1 piece)	3.0
Dates	30 g (1 oz)	2.5
Other:		
Baked beans	100 g (3½ oz)	5.0–8.5
Vegetables:		
Broad beans	100 g (3½ oz) boiled	4.2
Peanuts	30 g (1 oz)	2.5
Spinach	100 g (3½ oz)	6.3
Corn	100 g (3½ oz)	4.7
Cabbage	100 g (3½ oz)	2.5
Potato	100 g (3½ oz; 1 medium)	2.0

diets is a contributor to the increase in the 'diseases of civilization', particularly bowel disease. About 120 years ago, Western people changed from wholemeal to white bread and reduced the amount of vegetables and fruit they ate, replacing them with cakes, pastries and sweets. Following this dietary change, certain bowel diseases have been diagnosed more frequently. Appendicitis has increased in incidence, as has diverticular disease of the bowel (which now affects over 40 per cent of middle-aged people). Bowel cancer is increasing, as are intestinal polyps. Today more people develop haemorrhoids (piles), which affect one person in every four over the age of 50. Varicose veins are also more common, affecting 20 per cent of Western women compared with 4 per cent of African women.

The discomfort induced by the diseases and the frequency

Table 8.2: Calcium content of typical average servings of common foods

Food	Calcium (mg)	Serving size
Milk (whole or skimmed)	280	250 mL
Yoghurt	310	200 g
Swiss cheese	285	30 g
Cheddar cheese	260	30 g
Processed cheese	205	30 g
Cottage cheese	190	200 g
Canned salmon	110	¼ cup
Broccoli	60	60 g
Orange	60	150 g
Fish	50	100 g
Baked beans	40	100 g
Egg	30	55 g
Carrots	30	90 g
French beans	30	60 g
Bran flakes	20	30 g
Steak	20	100 g
Bread (slice)	10	25 g
Potato	10	(large)

Source: Dairy Corporation (NSW).

of the diseases themselves can be reduced, especially among menopausal and postmenopausal women, if people increase the quantity of fibre in their diet, so that they eat more than 30 g a day.

Increasing fibre in the diet

Eat more oatmeal (porridge) and wholegrain bread instead of white bread. This is important as fibre from cereals is better utilized than fibre from vegetables or fruit. But so that you eat a varied diet, choose green vegetables or fruit some days. On other days, you may choose to eat root vegetables or, if you like them, baked beans from time to time, as they are rich in fibre (Table 8.1). In other words, you should eat more grain cereal, vegetables and fruit (including the skins of apples and stone fruit) than you have been accustomed to eat, but less cakes, biscuits, sweets and sugar. If you can, you should eat 120 g (4 oz) or more of green, leafy vegetables or some fresh fruit every day.

Vitamins and minerals

If you eat a mixed diet, including fresh vegetables and fruit, you will probably obtain all the vitamins you need from your diet. However, you should increase the calcium-containing foods as at menopause calcium is less easily absorbed from the gut and, in consequence, more should be eaten. Lack of calcium is a factor leading to osteoporosis. Foods containing calcium are listed in Table 8.2 and you should make sure that you obtain 1500 mg of calcium a day. If you do not obtain this amount from food, you should take a calcium tablet every evening (see p. 87).

Avoiding bad food habits

You will feel healthier if you follow the recommendations just made, and if you can avoid the 'bad' food habits listed in Table 8.3.

OBESITY IN MIDDLE AGE

As was mentioned on p. 65, when women grow older they tend to put on weight. In the USA, an average white woman gains 10 kg (22 lbs) between the ages of 18 and 50. Surveys in Britain and the USA show that by the age of 50, one woman in

Table 8.3: Bad food habits

* Missing meals
* Replacing meals with snacks of poor nutritional quality, such as tea and sweet biscuits
* Constantly nibbling on lollies, sweet biscuits or cakes
* Not using enough milk or cheese
* Eating insufficient meat, fish, chicken or legumes (dried peas, beans, lentils)
* Drinking less than 1 litre (5 cups) of fluid daily
* Replacing meals with alcohol
* Shaking on large amounts of salt
* Unable to chew because of ill-fitting dentures or poor teeth
* Running out of basic groceries.

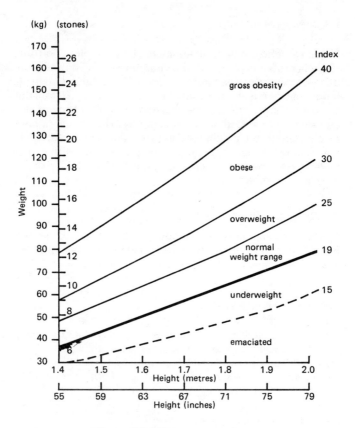

Figure 8.2: The body mass index

five is obese. Obesity is defined in several ways. The one that has proved the most accurate and the most useful is the Quetelet Index, or body mass index (BMI).

This index is calculated by measuring your weight in kilograms and your height in metres. The weight is then divided by the square of the height (Fig. 8.2). This produces a ratio. If your BMI is 30 or more, you are obese. The part of your body in which fat is deposited is important. If you deposit most of the fat on your trunk (your back, abdomen and waist), you are at greater risk of developing heart disease.

Obesity carries health hazards:

- High blood pressure is more common among obese people and if the woman loses weight, her blood pressure is often lowered.
- Stroke is twice as common.
- Heart disease is more common.
- Diabetes is five times as common and may be cured if the woman loses weight.
- Gall bladder disease is more common and more difficult to treat.
- Osteoarthritis, especially of the hips, knees and back, is more painful if the person is obese.
- Shortness of breath is more common.

For these reasons many menopausal women may wish to lose weight. Losing weight for a short time is relatively easy, but the lost weight is regained rapidly. What an obese person, who is motivated, should try to do is to lose weight slowly and when she reaches the weight she wants, to keep at this weight.

Losing weight permanently is much harder. If it was easy, the annual appearance of new books on 'How to lose weight', or the many magazine articles would not appear!

A nutritious weight-reducing diet

If you want to lose weight and to maintain your lower weight, you need to change your eating behaviour, so that you eat less permanently but still eat a nutritious diet.

It is easy to read a diet sheet, it is harder to keep to the diet. A diet that is easy to follow and relatively easy to adhere to is given in Table 8.4 on page 74.

How to keep to your chosen diet

- Make sure that your diet is palatable and as much like the diet of the rest of your family as you can make it. Unless it is sufficiently varied and tasty, you will become bored with it and will return to your old, familiar eating habits.
- Don't gorge by eating only one large meal a day. You will reduce to, and maintain, a weight in the normal range more easily if you eat several small meals spread through the day.

Table 8.4: A weight-reducing diet

Daily allowances of nutrients:

Wholemeal (or enriched bread)	3 slices	(50 g each)
Potatoes (boiled or baked)	100 g	(3½ oz)
or Rice (boiled)	60 g	(2 oz)
Milk (skimmed)	600 ml	(1 pint)
Low-fat spread	12 g	(1½ oz)

You should eat breakfast (when you may wish to choose from your fruit allowance) and two main meals each day.

Food choices:

Fruit One piece of fruit: apple; orange; half a grapefruit (with sugar); fresh orange juice or orange juice with no added sugar, 100 g; pears; plums; peaches or 100 g of melon. Bananas are NOT allowed.

Vegetables (2 portions a day are allowed)
Unlimited amounts: Asparagus; artichoke; beans (green); bean shoots; broccoli; brussel sprouts; cabbage; cauliflower; cucumber; celery; lettuce; mushrooms; mustard and cress; onions; spinach; silver beet

and

50 g of beans (butter, red, haricot); or 50 g of carrots; or of leeks; peas; parsnip; swedes; or turnip.

Poultry, meat, fish, cheese (one portion a day) Choose from:

	Poultry (remove skin), or game	60 g
or	Meat (lean, cut off fat, but still don't fry), minced beef, lean steak, lamb, pork, liver, kidney	60 g
or	Fatty fish (salmon, sardines, herrings, trout, mackerel)	60 g
or	Cheese (cheddar, camembert, Danish blue, etc.)	60 g
or	White fish or shellfish	60 g
or	Two eggs	
or	Cottage cheese	100 g

Tea, coffee, water, soda water in unlimited amounts.

You must avoid: sugar, sweets, chocolates, jams, honey, pastries and puddings, cakes and buns, ice-cream, canned fruits.

You should avoid alcoholic drinks, but if you can't, limit yourself each day to:

	Beer 250 ml (10 fluid oz)
or	Whisky 30 ml (1 fluid oz)
or	Wine 125 ml (5 fluid oz)

This diet will provide about 4.2 MJ (1200 kcals) a day and is well balanced in nutrients.

- Don't miss breakfast and don't eat your last meal late at night. The reason for eating several small meals rather than a single, large meal is that smaller meals, eaten at shorter intervals, induce a relatively greater production of body heat, which is then dissipated into the surrounding air. Body heat is produced using energy, and that is what you are trying to do — to use more energy than you ingest.
- Do try to eat your meals at approximately the same time each day. This has the psychological effect of helping you to control your feelings of hunger at times other than meal times.
- Don't raid the fridge between meals.
- Don't keep sweets or bars of chocolate in the house.
- Eat a nutritious diet from a variety of foods in the five food groups.
- Limit your consumption of alcohol. Older people metabolize alcohol less efficiently.

9

OSTEOPOROSIS

Osteoporosis is an example of a disease that may be preventable in many women if physicians and the public were better informed.

G Donald Whedon:
New England Journal of Medicine 1981

As a woman grows older, her bones become more brittle, and more likely to collapse or fracture. The most common bones first to collapse are those of the vertebrae, which make up the spine. In fact, the collapse is preceded by tiny fractures in the bone. These small fractures are usually painless, although if the process goes on for some time, a whole vertebra may collapse, becoming wedge shaped instead of cube shaped. This leads to the decrease in the person's height that is often observed among older women. About one woman in ten loses one-fifth of her height between the age of 50 and 70 years. The most common fractures that occur later, in older people, are those of the wrist and the hip joint. This is because these bones have to carry the most weight if a person slips or falls. A fracture is an acute, painful event, which needs immediate help.

Not only is bone mass lost as a person grows older, but the main constituent of bone, calcium, is also lost. Calcium is the substance that gives bone its strength and its rigidity. The decrease in the amount of bone mass, to a point where fractures become likely, is given the name of osteoporosis. In

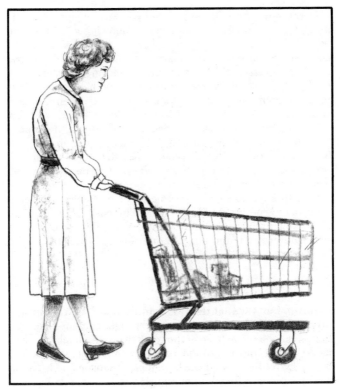

Figure 9.1: Dowager's hump

osteoporosis, the bone is brittle. Osteoporosis, to a greater or lesser extent, affects all old people, particularly women, but in only one-quarter does a dramatic event like a fracture of wrist or hip, or the collapse of a vertebra, occur.

Osteoporosis is not a new disease. It has been found in the skeletons of prehistoric people, in the bones of primitive people and among old people in both the developed and the developing nations. Because more people in the developed nations survive the hazards of disease in childhood, more people in these countries grow old, so that osteoporosis has become more common and now constitutes a major health problem.

In three-quarters of cases, osteoporosis develops silently, but, at an unexpected time, usually following a fall or some injury, the woman's forearm or her hip fractures. Vertebral collapse may also occur dramatically but usually the collapse slowly progresses, the woman suffering from increasing high back pain. In elderly women, the collapse of the vertebra leads to a bend in the back producing what has been called a Dowager's hump (Fig. 9.1). In some old women, several vertebrae collapse. The woman becomes shrunken, her upper body bent forward almost at a right angle to the ground, her head bent forward. In Europe from the 15th to the 18th centuries such women were often perceived to be witches and were hideously maltreated.

Osteoporosis is a disease of bone, or perhaps more accurately a degeneration of bone, which, in most cases, is due to the ageing process. To understand how the disease develops, the structure and functions of bone need to be discussed.

BONE

In November 1974, at the Hadar in Ethiopia, Don Johanson, driving slowly in a Land-Rover through ancient lake-side deposits, looked back along the track the four-wheel drive had made. Lying on the ground he saw a fragment of fossilized bone. Searching around the fragment, Johanson and his associates eventually found other bones from the same skeleton — a lower jaw, some ribs, part of a pelvis, a thigh bone, some vertebrae and fragments of shin bone.

Careful study of the bones showed that they were of a female, about 3 feet tall, who had walked upright and had died 3 million years ago. Johanson called her Lucy. She is one of our ancestors.

Paleoanthropologists, like Don Johanson and the Leakey family, are trying to piece together the anatomy and social behaviour of mankind's ancestors from fossilized bones — all that remains of the people who lived in an area such as the Hadar and on the shores of Lake Turkana, 3 million years ago.

From this, one might infer that bone is a static, stable tissue, and that once a person is adult, bone ceases to grow and change.

Nothing could be further from the truth. Bone is almost as dynamic as skin. Bone is constantly dying and being replaced. Bone is resilient and is constantly adjusting its structure to meet new stresses. In other words, it is remodelling. Bone has a remarkable plasticity. It has these properties because of its structure and its chemical composition. Its structure comprises a covering of membrane, called periosteum, under which lie numerous blood vessels. Directly beneath the periosteum, there is a dense outer layer of compact bone (the cortical layer), which varies in thickness in different bones. The stronger the bone has to be, the thicker is the compact layer. For this reason, the bones of the arms and legs have thick compact layers because of the stresses they undergo, when the muscles attached to them contract. The compact bone encloses a small meshwork of spongy bone, which is made up of fine spikes of bone carefully arranged in ties and struts to give the bone stability when it is stressed by crushing or tearing. This is the spongy or trabecular layer of bone (Fig. 9.2). Inside this layer of the bones of the legs and arms is a hollow space filled with bone marrow. The vertebrae, the neck of the femur and the wrists do not have the central hollow space. Instead it is filled with trabecular bone. The vertebrae

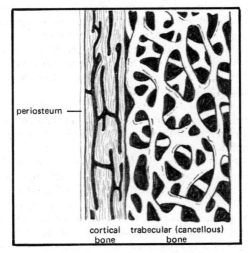

periosteum

cortical bone   trabecular (cancellous) bone

Figure 9.2: The structure of a long bone

differ from the long bones in another way. Although the spinal column, which is made up of vertebrae, carries the weight of the body and needs strength, the cortical layer of each vertebral bone is rather thin, the vertebra being made up mostly of spongy bone. However, the cubical shape of each vertebra gives strength to the spine without making it impossibly heavy.

The basic substance of bone is collagen. Both the compact and the spongy layers of bone are made up of special bone cells, which secrete the protein, collagen. Collagen is relatively plastic. To give bones rigidity and strength, it is impregnated (saturated) with lime salts, mainly calcium. If a piece of bone is placed in a weak acid solution, the calcium dissolves but the bone retains its shape, as this is dictated by the collagen framework. But now it can be twisted into knots or cut with a knife.

When a fragment of bone is examined under a microscope, its structure is shown. Compact bone consists of layers of collagen impregnated with calcium, rather like the coats of an

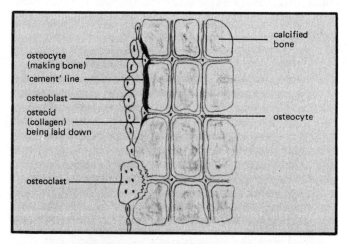

Figure 9.3: How bone is remodelled. Osteoblasts make osteoid and become enclosed in it to become osteocytes. The osteocytes together with osteoblasts (and probably osteoclasts) are involved in making calcified bone. The osteoclasts resorb calcified bone

onion (Fig. 9.3). Bone cells called osteoblasts produce collagen (which is also called osteoid). These cells lie in the bone between the periosteum and the compact bone. Other bone cells called osteocytes are also present and are found between the layers of bone, looking like plum stones. They are derived from some of the osteoblasts and may contribute to the strength of the bone. Osteoblasts (in association with cells called osteoclasts) cause calcium to be deposited through the collagen to produce a 'cement'. In the spongy layer the collagen has a different distribution, being laid down in a complicated manner, which may be described as a complex honeycomb (Fig. 9.4). The walls of the honeycomb are formed from collagen and impregnated with calcium, which gives the bone rigidity.

When bone dies or is changed in shape because of microscopic damage, or the need to adjust to new stresses on it, it is said to be remodelled. The remodelling of bone is going on all the time. Each year about 10 per cent of cortical bone and 40 per cent of trabecular bone is remodelled. Bone is first removed by the osteoclasts to a variable depth, depending on the particular bone being remodelled. The removal process (which takes about 2 weeks) ends when a line of tissue, con-

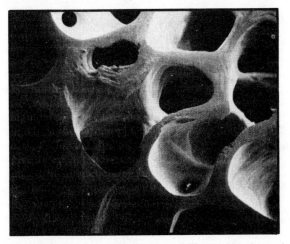

Figure 9.4: The structure of trabecular bone (courtesy of *Geriatrics* (USA))

sisting of collagen, and called the 'cement line', is laid down. On this cement line the osteoblasts lay down osteoid, which is then impregnated with calcium so that new bone is formed (Fig. 9.3). This process, which occurs in all parts of the bones, takes about 12 weeks in young people. As a person grows into late middle and old age, the process takes longer, less new osteoid being formed each day so that the process may take from 16 to 24 weeks to complete. During this time, in older people, the new osteoid formed is insufficient to replace completely the old bone that has been removed. At first, the young osteoclasts are beneficial, co-operating with osteoblasts to lay down calcium in the osteoid, which converts it into bone. Later the osteoclasts absorb bone, as just described.

This balanced process may become imbalanced in two ways. In the first way, the osteoblasts fail to make sufficient osteoid. The second way in which imbalance occurs is when the osteoblasts have a shortened life span, and die or are converted into osteoclasts before they have laid down much bone. If these changes occur, less bone is made than is removed and osteoporosis develops. As mentioned, these changes occur as a person grows older.

CALCIUM

Calcium has a major role in mediating the many vital functions of the cells that make up a human's body. To do this effectively the level of calcium ions in the blood and in fluid that surrounds the cells of the body has to be kept in a narrow range. Calcium ions are lost constantly in the urine but the body has mechanisms to maintain the level of calcium in the blood. This is done by hormones that increase the kidney's ability to resorb calcium that would otherwise be excreted in the urine, and increase absorption of dietary calcium from the gut. However, these mechanisms need to be protected. To do this the body has a calcium 'bank' from which calcium can be withdrawn urgently when needed, and into which calcium obtained from the diet can be repaid and deposited in the calcium bank. Bone fulfils the function of the calcium bank. In fact, bone is the body's only store of calcium. As well as being essential for vital cell functions, calcium gives rigidity and strength to bone, turning soft osteoid into firm bone. If a person fails to obtain enough calcium in the diet, or needs more calcium (which occurs as women grow older) or loses too much calcium in the urine, extra calcium is removed from the bones by the osteoclasts to keep up its concentration in the blood. This in turn leads to bone remodelling.

Calcification of bone is itself a complex process and depends on a variety of mechanisms.

How calcium is involved in bone formation

As has been mentioned, calcium (in the form of a compound called calcium hydroxyapatite) is deposited on the collagen and forms crystals, which give the bone its strength. Because bone is being remodelled constantly, calcium is released from the discarded bone and used to provide strength for the new bone. Each day about 700 g of calcium is exchanged between blood plasma and the bones. A small amount of calcium (about 150 mg) is excreted in the urine and is lost to the body, but at the same time calcium is obtained from the diet, which replaces the lost calcium.

An average European diet provides about 1100 mg of calcium each day, principally in milk and milk products such as cheese, and to a lesser extent in bread (which in England has calcium added to the flour to counteract the calcium-hoarding properties of a substance in the flour called phytate). The diet of most people in the hungry, developing world does not contain much milk. so that the amount of calcium provided is lower. In India, for example, an average of 50 mg per head per day is obtained, which is only about one-third of that provided by a European diet.

This is not such a serious situation as it might appear. Between 60 and 70 per cent of the 1100 mg of calcium in the European diet is not available for absorption. This is related in part to Western diet, which is rich in protein and high in salt, two substances that hold calcium, preventing it being absorbed. The calcium that is not absorbed is lost in the faeces. A much lower proportion of the calcium in the Indian diet is 'held' and then lost in the faeces so that relatively more is available to be absorbed. In both diets, in general, sufficient calcium is provided by food and is absorbed to replace that lost to the body.

The calcium is absorbed through the cells lining the intestine by becoming bound to protein-carriers, which transport it from the gut into the blood. Before this can happen, there must be a certain amount of vitamin D_3 in the body, as the protein is unable to link to calcium in the absence of this vitamin. When vitamin D_3 is deficient, rickets occurs in children, and the bones of adults become soft and distorted.

The absorbed calcium is transported in the blood and transferred to the bones or, if the blood level becomes too high, is excreted by the kidneys. Although the limits of the amount of calcium in the blood are strictly regulated, a constant exchange occurs from the calcium in the diet into the blood, from the blood to the bones, from the bones to the blood, from the blood to the kidneys, from the kidneys to the urine, and from the urine back into the blood or out into the lavatory pan.

The regulation of this sequence is complex, and scientists are still discovering more about how it operates. Once the calcium has been absorbed into the blood stream, the regulation of its level in the blood is controlled by two hormones. The first is a hormone produced by tiny glands found in the neck near the thyroid gland. They are called parathyroid glands and the hormone they produce is called parathyroid hormone. If the blood level of calcium falls, more parathyroid hormone is secreted. This mobilizes calcium from the bones, and by stimulating vitamin D_3 production in the kidneys reduces the amount lost in the urine. The second hormone involved in regulating the level of calcium in the blood is produced by the thyroid gland and is called calcitonin. Although calcitonin is known to be involved in regulating calcium in bone, how it is involved is unknown despite intense research.

These complex interactions could cause problems if anything went wrong, but, at least up to the time of the menopause, in healthy people they rarely do. This is because sufficient calcium is obtained from food to keep the blood levels normal without drawing on the calcium stores in bone. At night a slight problem arises, as most people sleep, not snack, at night. As calcium continues to be lost in the urine, its level in the blood would drop if the parathyroid hormone didn't come into play by removing a small amount of calcium from bone. But the calcium is replaced the next day from the diet.

Two other groups of hormones are also involved in regulating the loss of calcium from bone. These are the sex hormones. In women the sex hormones, oestrogen and progesterone, are produced by the ovaries. In men the sex hormone androgen is produced by the testicles.

The sex hormones protect the bones from the calcium-extracting effect of parathyroid hormone in at least two ways. First, oestrogen is involved in the synthesis of vitamin D_3, which in turn increases the amount of calcium absorbed from the gut. Second, oestrogen either directly or indirectly increases the secretion of calcitonin.

In most people the system works admirably. The bones, which are constantly being renewed, remain strong and rigid. The diet provides all the calcium needed to keep them strong; there is enough vitamin D_3 to ensure that calcium in the diet is absorbed; parathyroid hormone and calcitonin regulate the level in the body. But certain things can upset this admirable state of affairs. One is reduced mobility; another is the loss or reduction of the sex hormones.

Reduced mobility leads to a loss of calcium from bone but the effect of the loss of, or reduction in, oestrogen is much more serious.

As we discussed earlier, the level of oestrogen in the blood falls dramatically after the menopause. When this happens, first, less calcium is absorbed from the food eaten and second, the level of calcitonin may fall. The result of these two changes is that to keep up the level of calcium in the blood, the parathyroid hormone takes over to mobilize calcium from the bones, with the result that over a period of time bone tissue is resorbed. This leads to a reduction in the bone mass.

CHANGES IN BONE MASS WITH AGEING

Until the age of 35, bone mass increases (Table 9.1). It then stabilizes for a few years, after which the bone mass begins to

Table 9.1: Changes in bone mass with ageing

Bone loss occurs when resorption exceeds formation

Trabecular bone (vertebrae, neck femur, lower end radius)
Gain till age 35–40
Loss from age 40–45 onwards:

40–50	0.5–1.0% per annum
50–60	3.0–5.0% per annum in women
60+	0.5–1.0% per annum

Cortical bone (long bones of arms and legs)
Gain till age 35–40
Loss from age 40–45 onwards — ? a steady loss at
0.5–1.0% per annum

decrease. Over an average lifetime of 75 years, a woman may lose about 25 to 35 per cent of her cortical bone, which is the major component of the bones of the arms and legs. Over the same lifetime, a woman may lose 40 to 50 per cent of her spongy (trabecular) bone. Because men produce the male sex hormone androgen into old age, they are luckier, losing only about two-thirds of women's bone loss.

Bone loss does not occur at a regular rate and, as well, the proportion of bone lost varies between individuals. The effect of the bone loss also varies — the more bone originally, the fewer will be the clinical effects of osteoporosis.

There is some controversy about the rate of bone loss from trabecular and from cortical bone. This is because different methods of estimating bone loss give different results.

The consensus is that trabecular bone begins to be lost from about the age of 35. The loss is mainly from the vertebrae, the wrists and the lower jaw. At first the rate of loss is slow, averaging 0.5 per cent of trabecular bone mass each year. Once a woman reaches the menopause, the rate of trabecular bone loss increases to between 3 and 5 per cent a year. This rate of bone loss persists for 5 to 10 years after which the rate slows to between 0.5 and 1 per cent. Cortical bone loss starts about a decade later than trabecular bone loss, at the age of 45 in both sexes. The initial rate of loss is 0.3 to 0.5 per cent each year. In women the rate of loss increases to 2 to 3 per cent in the 5 to 10 years after the menopause, and then the rate decreases to 0.3 to 0.5 per cent a year.

Not all women lose bone at the same rate. A Swiss study of 35 women followed for 3 years after their menopause showed that half of them did not lose bone; a quarter lost between 1 and 2 per cent of their bone mass, and a quarter lost larger amounts (up to 14 per cent) of their bone mass. The women who lost bone had phases when relatively little bone was lost, followed by phases of increased bone loss.

The reasons for the different rates of bone loss are not clear, but studies show that women who are thin, who smoke, who consume alcohol heavily, who are prescribed certain drugs and whose calcium intake from food is low, may lose bone at a greater rate and may be more likely to develop the clinical signs of osteoporosis.

Men have a larger bone mass and do not experience the hormonal changes of the menopause. Consequently they do not have the increased rate of bone loss until the age of 70. After the age of 70 the pattern of bone loss changes. Men and women now lose bone at an equal rate. When the density of the bone falls below a critical level, fractures occur. The vertebrae are affected particularly and 'wedge' fractures become common. The collapse of the vertebra leads to the 'Dowager's hump' (See Fig. 9.1). Fracture of the hip is increasingly common with ageing and because women have lost more bone before the age of 70 than men, twice as many elderly women fracture their hips compared with men.

WHAT LEADS TO OSTEOPOROSIS?

At present the reason why older people, especially women, develop osteoporosis is also not clear. Several factors have been suggested. These include:
- reduced levels of sex hormones
- taking less exercise
- reduced calcium intake or absorption
- smoking
- ? increased tea or coffee consumption (by increasing calcium loss in the urine)
- ? increased alcohol consumption.

Reduced levels of sex hormones   During the reproductive

years, at least until the menopause, oestrogen produced by
the woman's ovaries prevents bone loss. The effect of oestrogen is indirect because no 'receptors' for oestrogen have
been found in bone. (There may be receptors on the osteoblasts.) This means that oestrogen acts by suppressing the
activity of bone-resorbing hormones, such as the parathyroid
gland hormone; or by increasing the effect of calcitonin, or by
increasing the quantity of calcium absorbed from the gut; or
by reducing the loss of calcium in the urine. The decline in the
level of oestrogen circulating in the blood, which occurs at
and after the menopause, seems to be the major factor leading
to osteoporosis in women.

Reduced calcium intake and absorption   The strength and
rigidity of bone is dependent on calcium salts being deposited
on the meshwork of collagen that makes up bone. As people
grow older, they absorb less dietary calcium from their gut;
and women who have osteoporosis tend to absorb less than
other women of a similar age. As was discussed earlier, a negative calcium balance (more calcium lost to the body in the
urine and faeces than is absorbed from food or calcium supplements) will lead to osteoporosis.

A further factor is that postmenopausal women need to
absorb twice as much calcium to prevent deficiency, compared with younger women or men. The reason for this is
complex and may be related to the reduction in oestrogen
circulating in a woman's body after the menopause.

To remain in calcium balance, a woman who is postmenopausal needs to take 1500 mg of calcium a day in her food or as
a calcium supplement.

With these facts known, it is unfortunate that many menopausal women reduce their intake of dairy foods (milk and
cheese).

Reduced mobility   Middle-aged people, especially women,
tend to take less exercise than when they were younger and
this is one of the factors that over the years may lead to osteoporosis, as exercise is known to increase the amount of calcium in the bones. The loss of bone in middle-aged women
may be greater than that of middle aged men, because women
lack androgen — the male sex hormone — which is thought to

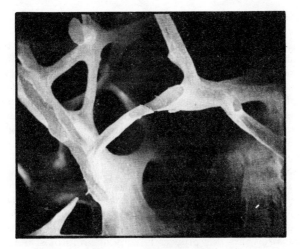

Figure 9.5: The structure of osteoporotic bone
— compare with Figure 9.4
(courtesy of *Geriatrics* (USA))

protect against bone loss. Androgen secretion is increased by exercise and this may be one way in which exercise helps to prevent osteoporosis.

Smoking   There is evidence that women who smoke have an earlier menopause and that osteoporosis occurs earlier and is more severe if the woman smokes. This is because smoking in some way increases the metabolism of the sex hormones by the liver so that a lower level of circulating oestrogen is available to prevent bone loss.

Increased ingestion of caffeine and alcohol   Some studies suggest that an increased ingestion of caffeine is a factor in the development of osteoporosis by increasing the loss of calcium in the urine. Middle-aged women tend to drink more tea and coffee than younger women, and a few drink more alcohol. However, it has not been proved that the increased caffeine and alcohol increase the likelihood of developing osteoporosis.

THE SYMPTOMS OF OSTEOPOROSIS

In itself, bone loss in most women is symptomless, but if an accident occurs, such as a fall, the weakened bone may break or collapse. Within a community, the frequency with which bone fractures occur gives some indication of the size of the problem of osteoporosis. In the USA, for example, osteoporosis is responsible for over one million bone fractures each year, and the costs (direct and indirect) of caring for osteoporosis sufferers have been estimated as $6 billion; in Australia the cost exceeds $250 million.

The bones that make up the spinal column, the vertebrae, are most frequently affected. In most women over the age of 50, vertebral bones become slowly, insidiously brittle (Fig. 9.5). Over this period, it is likely that tiny fractures occur in some of the slender ties and struts that make up spongy bone. For many years this process is without symptoms, but the woman gradually loses height and may develop a 'Dowager's hump'. The loss in height may be small, but one woman in eight loses 20 per cent of her height between the age of 50 and 70. In a few women the bone loss from the vertebrae leads to a sudden complete collapse of a vertebra — a compression fracture. This is accompanied by severe back pain. The compression fracture may be initiated by a routine activity such as bending, rising from a chair or bed or lifting an object.

But in most women, the vertebral compression occurs without symptoms and leads to a reduction in the woman's height. In the most severe cases the woman's back becomes bent and she develops a 'witch like' posture. This occurs in about three women in every hundred between the age of 40 and 60 and in seven women in every hundred over the age of 60.

Two other fractures occur increasingly with age and both are more common in women than in men (at least before the age of 80). Studies in Sweden in the 1960s and in the USA in the 1980s show that fractures of the lower end of the forearm (Colles fracture) and the hip increase as a person ages (Figure 9.6). Most hip fractures occur after the age of 70 in both sexes. Over the age of 75, one woman in every three and one of every six men will sustain a hip fracture. Hip fractures are disabling,

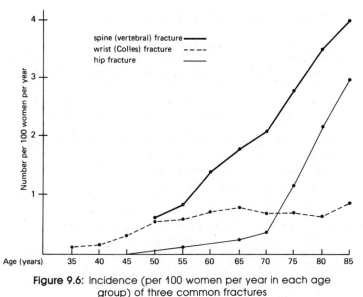

Figure 9.6: Incidence (per 100 women per year in each age group) of three common fractures

costly to treat and often life threatening. In 1980, in the USA, 230 000 elderly people had a hip fracture. Of these people, one in ten died within six months and between a quarter and a half were never able to walk or to function as well. Many of these elderly people had to remain in nursing homes permanently.

The incidence of hip fractures also has been increasing in Britain in the past decade, as studies from Nottingham show. The studies confirm that men and women over the age of 65 are at the greatest risk, and that in each age group after 65 years, women are at greater risk than men. About 50 000 people in Britain fracture a hip each year.

Taken together, collapse of a vertebra or the fracture of the forearm or the hip affect about one woman in four over the age of 60. Although all women lose bone, only 25 per cent develop symptomatic osteoporosis.

PREVENTING OSTEOPOROSIS

Prevention is crucial as few treatments significantly increase bone mass once it is lost and when they do, they predominantly affect trabecular (spongy) bone mass, sometimes at the expense of cortical (the solid) bone mass.

C. N. de Deuxchaisnes, 1983

Despite the lack of scientific evidence that osteoporosis can be prevented, the interplay of various factors discussed provides a rational basis for treatment that may delay, or prevent, osteoporosis (Table 9.2). It is one that every woman can follow.

Table 9.2: Possible ways to prevent or delay osteoporosis

* Take ½ to 1 hour of exercise three times a week
* Take 1.5 g of calcium each day as dairy products or a calcium tablet
* Reduce or stop cigarette smoking
* Limit the amount of alcohol you take
* Discuss with a doctor whether or not to take small daily doses of oestrogens (and progestogens) at least for the first 5 to 10 years after your menopause
* Avoid taking barbiturates as they seem to increase the fracture rate

Calcium intake

As the bones increase in density from the age of 12 to about the age of 35, this is a period during which calcium intake should be kept high. Young people, especially women, should make sure that they obtain at least 800 mg of calcium in their daily diet. This amount can be obtained from about 750 ml of milk (whole or skimmed) or 90 g of cheese (Table 9.3).

Women from about the age of 35 should make sure that they increase their calcium intake in an effort to counteract the osteoporotic process. From the time of the menopause an increased calcium intake is probably even more important. Peri- and postmenopausal women should ingest at least 1500 mg of calcium a day.

Table 9.3: Calcium content of typical average servings of common foods

Food	Calcium (mg)	Serving size
Milk (whole or skimmed)	280	250 mL
Yoghurt	310	200 g
Swiss cheese	285	30 g
Cheddar cheese	260	30 g
Processed cheese	205	30 g
Cottage cheese	190	200 g
Canned salmon	110	¼ cup
Broccoli	60	60 g
Orange	60	150 g
Fish	50	100 g
Baked beans	40	100 g
Egg	30	55 g
Carrots	30	90 g
French beans	30	60 g
Bran flakes	20	30 g
Steak	20	100 g
Bread (slice)	10	25 g
Potato	10	(large)

Source: Dairy Corporation (NSW).

Skimmed milk provides 1 mg of calcium per millilitre and 90 g of cheese contains around 800 mg of calcium. If a woman prefers not to eat dairy products, she can buy calcium supplements. Argument, among specialist physicians, continues about which is the most effective calcium preparation. But it is agreed that at least some calcium should be taken in the evening, as the greatest loss of calcium from bone occurs during sleep. Controversy and debate, often heated and emotional, continues between groups of doctors who are involved in osteoporosis research, whether calcium has any protective value in preventing osteoporosis. There appears to be no consensus. However, a lack of calcium in the diet leads to osteoporosis in animals, and it seems sensible to recommend that menopausal women should take calcium tablets or eat calcium-containing foods.

Sex hormones, particularly oestrogen

At least there is agreement about oestrogen. All experts agree that small daily doses of oestrogen will reduce bone loss from the vertebrae and probably the long bones of women who have passed the menopause. The most recent, carefully designed study about the effect of oestrogen was reported in 1987 in California. Dr Ettinger and his colleagues found the height of postmenopausal women who took small doses of oestrogen each day did not decrease and their risk of developing a fracture of a vertebra was half that of women who did not take oestrogen. The risk of a wrist fracture was halved and that of a hip fracture reduced two and a half times.

However, oestrogens given to postmenopausal women have been implicated in the development of uterine cancer, and care has to be taken to choose a dose that will inhibit vertebral bone loss (and may promote bone formation) but will not increase the risk of cancer.

Research since 1980 has shown that the dose of oestrogen is critical. A daily dose of 0.02 mg of ethinyl oestradiol will not restore any bone loss that has already occurred but will inhibit further bone loss. A dose of more than 0.025 mg of ethinyl oestradiol may lead to a net gain of bone. Any of the other oestrogens may be chosen in place of ethinyl oestradiol and, in equivalent doses, will have the same effect on bone. However, the higher the dose of oestrogen, the greater the risk of stimulation of the cells of the endometrium and possible development of uterine cancer, so a balance has to be struck. The possible dangerous side effects of oestrogen are reduced if progestogen is given as well, for 14 days in every 30.

When oestrogen and progestogen are given together, oestrogen should prevent most of the loss of bone, while progestogen may produce some formation of bone with the result that the total bone mass may increase, which would be of value in preventing osteoporosis. Some scientists believe that a progestogen given alone will also retard bone loss; others deny that the hormone has any effect.

Another interesting observation was made. If oestrogen (in a dose of 0.01 mg of ethinyl oestradiol or equivalent) was given together with calcium, this lower dose was effective in preventing significant bone loss from the spine and the long bones of the body. Recently, some doubt has been expressed that the combination of oestrogen and calcium has any benefit over that of oestrogen alone.

At present, it is uncertain if a postmenopausal woman needs to take oestrogen and progestogen for the rest of her life or only for 5 to 10 years after the menopause, when bone loss is greatest. Most opinion holds that 5 to 10 years is sufficient, but that calcium should be continued for life in one form or another.

Should all or only certain women take oestrogen? As oestrogen reduces or prevents bone loss, especially from the vertebrae, should all or only some women take oestrogen? Recently it has become possible to measure accurately the density of cortical bone in the forearm, and to relate this to the probable density of the vertebrae. Some investigators have found the relationship close, others say that the forearm reading is of little value in determining the density of the trabecular bones of the spine.

This problem may be overcome by measuring spinal density with a computerised tomographic (CAT) scanner; or by using a technique of dual-photon absorbiometry. Both techniques are expensive.

Preliminary studies have shown that vertebral fracture is unlikely to occur if the spinal trabecular bone density is above a certain level. Women with the higher bone density need not take oestrogen. But to detect this group of women, all menopausal women would have to be 'screened' for reduced bone density, which would be a major administrative and costly exercise, particularly as the screening would need to be made at least five times over a period of 5 to 7 years. Even then the results would be unpredictable as regards the chance of fracture later on. It also could cause considerable anxiety to a woman to be told that she has a bone mass below the average for her age, even though it might be above that likely to be associated with a fracture.

In a consensus discussion held in late 1986, three leading US experts on osteoporosis agreed that routine screening of all menopausal women is neither cost-effective nor benefits individual women in any way. Against this a group of Australian scientists argue that although screening for reduced bone density in the spine would be prohibitively costly, an estimate of the density of the bone of the forearm 'would give as much information about spinal osteoporosis as the

expensive measurement of the spine'. Other scientists dis-
agree, claiming that forearm bone density is only closely
related to fractures of the forearm and hip. These fractures are
only one-tenth as common as spine fractures, at least before
the age of 70, and only occur as the result of a fall.

Further research should resolve this matter.

Exercise

First, the amount of exercise taken daily should be increased.
The exercise need not be strenuous, but should be sufficient
to put 'stress' on the spine and the legs. A brisk walk or rather
energetic gardening are as beneficial as any other kind of
exercise. Exercise should be taken for half to one hour three
times a week. Evidence from the USA and from Australia
shows that this amount of exercise, over a period of a year,
increased the bone mass (determined by measuring the total
amount of calcium in the body) of menopausal women by 2.5
per cent, while a 'control group' of similar age, eating habits
and socioeconomic status, who were sedentary, had lost 2.5
per cent of their total bone mass by the end of the year.

Other drugs

Several other drugs have been suggested as helping to prevent
osteoporosis. One is fluoride. Fluoride certainly thickens the
compact area of long bone, which may add to its strength. In
spongy bone, the honeycomb ties and struts are also thickened, but paradoxically this may make them less able to resist
twisting stresses. Vitamin D_3 (either natural or synthetic)
helps to increase the absorption and transport of calcium but
is only needed in people who are deficient in vitamin D_3

Androgens or anabolic testosterone have been suggested as
an alternative to oestrogen treatment. The argument is that
men, who secrete testosterone, lose bone more slowly than
women, and that therefore androgens protect against bone
loss. However, careful investigations show that androgens are
less effective than oestrogens in reducing bone loss and may
cause liver damage.

Combinations of the above drugs, together with calcium
have also been recommended. Once again, the benefits are

doubtful, and there is no evidence, at present, that any of the above drugs alone, or in combination, reduce the fracture rate in elderly women.

Calcitonin

Despite intensive research since 1960, the role of calcitonin in regulating bone formation and resorption is still unclear. Very big doses of calcitonin suppress bone resorption in artificial conditions, but reduced levels of 'active' calcitonin have not been found in the blood of women who have osteoporosis. Recent research suggests that daily injections of calcitonin are as effective as oestrogen in preventing bone loss, but are much more expensive. Calcitonin may be of use to prevent osteoporosis in women who cannot take oestrogen preparations.

THE TREATMENT OF ESTABLISHED, DEFORMING OSTEOPOROSIS

There is no treatment that is able to restore bone loss to normal, particularly in women over the age of 70, when osteoporosis is often first diagnosed because of a fracture or a deformity of the spine. The measures mentioned in the prevention of progressive bone loss should be used, and, in addition, elderly women may benefit from vitamin D, fluoride, anabolic steroids, or combinations of the above drugs to improve bone formation. There is no scientific evidence that the above drugs, including the sex hormones, have any real benefit, and well designed trials are needed to determine their value.

10

THE MENOPAUSE AND BODY SYSTEMS

In this chapter we shall consider the relationships between the menopause and the heart, the urinary tract and the breasts.

THE HEART

It has been believed for some decades that oestrogen produced by the ovaries protects women during their reproductive years against heart disease. This belief is based, first, on the observation that heart attacks occur four times as often among young men as among young women. After the menopause the difference decreases, so that by the age of 60, men are only twice as likely to have heart attacks as women. The second observation is that women who have an early menopause, either following surgical removal of the ovaries or naturally, have twice the risk of having a heart attack in the following years. These findings can be interpreted to suggest that if an oestrogen is prescribed to women after the menopause, they will be protected to some extent against the risk of heart disease.

The factors that increase the risk of heart disease have been investigated by many medical scientists, and no real consensus has been reached. Most agree that several risk factors are involved and the more risk factors that a person has the greater is the chance of a heart attack. The factors are: the amount of fat in the diet, cigarette smoking, lack of exercise, high blood pressure (often associated with obesity) and diabetes. The first of the risk factors has received the most attention.

The more fat eaten in the diet the greater is the risk of coronary heart disease. Fats are taken up from the intestines, enter the blood stream and are transported around the body. Fats are made up of several different substances. Those important in the development of heart disease are saturated fatty acids and cholesterol. Of the two, the level of cholesterol in the blood has been shown to be related to the risk of heart disease. Cholesterol is transported in the blood attached to fatty substances called lipoproteins. In many medical centres, middle-aged people are advised to have an annual blood test to measure their levels of plasma cholesterol, and those with raised levels are advised to alter their diet and to exercise more. Recently the measurements have become more sophisticated. It has been found that lipoprotein–cholesterol is not a single substance, but can be divided into fractions, depending on the density of the lipoprotein. The most important of these are: high density lipoprotein–cholesterol (HDL–C); low density lipoprotein–cholesterol (LDL–C); and very low density lipoprotein–cholesterol (VDL–C). When the level of these subgroups was correlated with the risk of heart disease, it became apparent that a rise in LDL–cholesterol increased the risk of a heart attack, while a rise in HDL–cholesterol decreased the risk, although only slightly.

Most doctors now measure total plasma cholesterol, and if this is raised they measure the subgroups HDL–C and LDL–C, which together carry over 90 per cent of the cholesterol in the blood.

It is known that the level of LDL–C increases with age, although less in women than men. It also increases with obesity, and diminishes if the diet contains more complex carbohydrates and fibre and less saturated fats ('the prudent diet'). HDL–C increases if a 'prudent diet' is eaten, if weight is reduced, if exercise is taken regularly and the person ceases to smoke.

Because of concern that the sex hormones might influence HDL–C and LDL–C, several investigations have been made among menopausal women.

The research has shown that oestrogen given alone to women who have had their ovaries removed (oöphorectomy) or to postmenopausal women, leads to a reduction in LDL–C, and a small rise in HDL–C. The changes are not marked, and all that can be said is that oestrogens given to menopausal women do not *increase* the risk of heart disease. Because of the many variables affecting the risk (smoking, weight, diet, life-style), it cannot be said that oestrogen replacement *protects* a woman against ischaemic heart disease.

The effect of sex steroids treatment on the woman's blood lipids is complicated by the fact that it is now usual to give a progestogen for at least 12 days each month in addition to oestrogen when treating menopausal symptoms.

The question that now has to be answered is: 'Do progestogens affect blood lipids, and is the lipid level influenced by the type of progestogen and the dose prescribed?'

The results from many studies are inconsistent and confusing, partly because in the investigations larger doses of progestogen were given than are prescribed today and partly because of flawed methodology.

Study of the available papers suggests that addition of a progestogen (in the larger doses then prescribed) for 10 to 14 days a month has only a slight effect on blood lipids, leading to a small but inconsistent increase in LDL and a small, inconsistent, reduction in HDL. There seems little difference in the effects of the three most often prescribed progestogens (norethisterone, norgestrel, medroxyprogesterone acetate), but in one study the last two had a slightly lesser effect on blood fats. As mentioned on p. 50, the new generation progestogens, which have no effect on blood lipids, will probably replace the above three progestogens currently prescribed in sequential oestrogen–progestogen preparations (hormone replacement therapy).

The beneficial alterations in the blood lipid levels of postmenopausal women due to oestrogen suggested to some doctors that if menopausal women were prescribed oestrogen they would be protected against heart attacks. What is the evidence that this idea is true?

There are several bits of information available. The first is that a randomized trial in which men who had had a heart attack were given oestrogen or a placebo, had to be stopped because the men taking oestrogen did not have fewer heart attacks than the men taking a placebo, but did have an increased chance of venous thrombosis and pulmonary embolism. Second, one study showed that more heart attacks occurred in women over 35 who were taking the pill than in women using other forms of contraception. However, in this study oestrogen was a lesser risk factor than smoking. Third, in two studies of menopausal women who had had heart attacks, the chance of having another heart attack was neither increased, nor decreased, among women taking oestrogen. Against this, two American studies have found that postmenopausal oestrogen therapy is associated with a *reduced risk* of heart attacks.

Another recent study has suggested that oestrogen given to women after the menopause may *increase* the risk of heart disease and stroke. The Director of the study, Dr William Castelli, believes that his findings, which contradict earlier studies, is due to the fact that in the other studies, the women's risk of heart disease occurring before they took oestrogen was not assessed. Dr Castelli found that women who take oestrogen have a 60 per cent greater risk of developing heart disease and stroke than women not prescribed oestrogen.

However, another study published in the same medical journal on the same date suggested that oestrogen decreased the risk of heart attack.

The publication of these two papers led to a series of letters that were printed in the same journal. The letters made it clear that there is a considerable difference of opinion about the benefit or lack of benefit of oestrogens in reducing heart attacks in older women. What is needed is a careful clinical trial to find the answer. It would be very expensive and probably difficult to arrange.

The conflicting evidence led the National Institute of Health in the USA to convene a conference in 1984 to discuss whether oestrogen therapy reduced or increased the chance of a heart attack. The conference reported that 'there is no conclusive evidence that oestrogen therapy has a role in the prevention of heart disease or that postmenopausal women receiving oestrogen therapy are at an increased risk of heart disease'.

A study published in 1987 supports this statement. It showed that women who had a natural menopause, whether they had taken oestrogen or not after the menopause, had no increased risk of coronary heart disease. But women who had had their ovaries removed before the time of the natural menopause, and had not been prescribed oestrogen, had an increased risk of heart attack. If they were prescribed oestrogen, the increased risk was prevented.

THE URINARY TRACT SYSTEM

Women are more likely to develop urinary symptoms than men. About 20 per cent of women aged between 20 and 50 are likely to have an attack of painful and frequent urination in any year, indicating a probable attack of cystitis.

Many women have involuntary urinary leakage. The leakage may occur following sneezing, coughing, laughing or excitement, or may follow an uncontrollable urge to pass urine. The proportion of women who have involuntary leakage of urine (urinary incontinence) in an inappropriate place more than twice a month, increases from less than 5 per cent in women under the age of 35 to over 15 per cent in women over the age of 60, according to a survey made in England.

Another study made in Sweden, of women over the age of 70, found that 40 per cent of the women had some degree of incontinence, and it was sufficiently severe to make life unpleasant in half of these. Most of the women had managed to cope and had not sought medical help.

In the Netherlands, a study of 700 postmenopausal women in a medium-sized town showed that 27 per cent had urinary incontinence.

There are several varieties of urinary incontinence. Some women who have infection of the bladder are incontinent. Other women have 'stress' incontinence, which is due to an anatomical failure of the muscles around the outlet of the bladder to close, particularly when the woman is 'stressed', for example when she laughs or jumps. Other incontinent women have so-called 'urgency' incontinence. This is due to an overactive bladder, which contracts when it contains only a small amount of urine. Other women have a mixture of stress incontinence and urgency incontinence. In fact, nearly two-thirds of the Dutch women who reported having urinary incontinence had the mixed type.

The diagnosis may be made easily or may require special tests to be made. Obviously urinary tract infection must be excluded and many women require urodynamic studies to identify the precise reason for the incontinence. In general, the treatment of stress incontinence is surgery, while urgency incontinence is treated by 'retraining' the bladder and taking drugs.

Recent reports from Europe suggest that vaginally administered oestrogen should be tried in postmenopausal women who complain of urinary incontinence, before surgery is contemplated or drugs given.

THE BREASTS

Following the menopause, the glandular tissues of the breast decrease in size, as they are no longer stimulated by oestrogen in the way that they were during the reproductive years. Often the breasts become smaller. In some women the breasts remain the same size or become larger because fat is deposited in the breasts.

Although the glandular tissue of the breast becomes relatively inactive after the menopause, breast cancer may develop in it. Breast cancer is the most common site of cancer in women. One woman in every 15 will develop breast cancer some time in her life, usually after the age of 50.

Breast cancer can only be cured if it is detected at an early stage. For this reason some form of breast examination at regular intervals has been recommended for all women, especially those nearing the menopause, and those in their postmenopausal years.

There are three ways of examining the breasts — breast self examination, breast examination by a doctor and mammography.

Breast self examination (BSE)

In the past 30 years the notion has arisen that if a woman examined her breasts each month from about the age of 25, any lump that had developed would be detected early. If the lump turned out to be a breast cancer, the early detection would lead to a better chance of cure.

Table 10.1: Guidelines for detecting breast cancer

* If a woman detects a lump in her breast she should see a doctor urgently so that its nature can be determined.
* A woman who has no breast problems and who is aged 25 or older should examine her breasts every month following a menstrual period or if she has reached the menopause every month about the same time.
* A woman who has no breast problems and who is aged 35 should have her breasts examined by a doctor every 3 years; and women over the age of 40 should have an annual breast examination.
* A woman who has no breast symptoms and who is aged 35 to 40 years should have a 'base line' mammogram, with which subsequent mammograms can be compared.
* A woman who has no breast symptoms and who is aged between 40 and 50 should consult with her doctor about the need for an annual mammogram. For example, women who have a mother or a sister who has had breast cancer, or who are childless or whose first child was born after the age of 35, probably should have annual mammograms from the age of 40.
* A woman who has no breast problems and who is aged 50 and over should have a mammogram each year.

Most national cancer societies have promoted breast self examination (BSE) as have many doctors and some women's groups. For example the Boston Women's Health Collective in their book: *The New Our Bodies: Ourselves*, wrote that they believe that women are the best monitors of their own breasts and probably will be able to detect an abnormality better than many doctors who have to take into account the wide variation in the breasts of different women, which they examine only once or twice a year. Women are also concerned that 'most doctors are trained to discredit what patients, particularly women, report about themselves'.

Studies by doctors about the value of BSE have been few and have been retrospective, that is they have asked women who have developed breast cancer whether they practised BSE or not, or have checked whether BSE increased the survival rate of women who had breast cancer. The results of these studies show that BSE is less effective in the early detection of breast cancer than examination by a trained doctor or by mammography.

Those who oppose BSE believe that the 'costs' of the procedure in terms of anxiety and possible unnecessary operations exceed the benefits. One such critic of BSE is Dr Francis Moore of the Harvard Medical School. In 1978 he wrote that he was worried about the 'millions of women nervously palpating their breasts in front of a mirror in response to subway advertisements, Cancer Society commercials, television and books published by the lay public'. Dr Moore is critical of books written by physicians that speak directly to the public. He writes 'such books go over the head of scientific data or literature and with paternalistic zeal tell the patients what to do, how to do it, what to think, how to rearrange prejudices and what kinds of doctors to consult'. He believes that breast self examination has not been proved to be of value and implies that it would be preferable if every woman's breasts were examined regularly by a doctor or a trained registered nurse.

Dr Moore is not alone in his criticism. The English medical journal, *The Lancet*, printed a review by two Canadian physicians in 1985. Their conclusions were that BSE might do more harm than good, especially in women under the age of 40, whose breasts respond more readily to the fluctuating hormone levels that occur during the menstrual cycle, and may develop transient breast lumps. If a lump is discovered, investigations including breast biopsy are usually necessary and may cause needless anxiety.

As a woman reaches her menopausal years the chance of developing breast cancer increases to about 2 per 1000 women each year. In this age group, BSE may have a benefit, but most women are reluctant to learn how to examine their breasts, and other techniques for breast examination are available.

However, some women may wish to practise BSE. You can do it if you follow these steps (provided by the Anti Cancer Council of Victoria).

Step 1 Stand in front of a mirror, put your hands by your side and look at your breasts. Then raise your hands above your head and look again. Now put your hands on your hips, press firmly, elbows forward (which puts the chest [pectoral] muscles on a stretch), and look again. You are looking at your breasts to see if the shape of each has changed since your last self examination; if any part of the skin is puckered; if there is a bulge or a flattened area in the breast; or if either nipple has been drawn into the breast tissue.

Step 2: Getting into position If your breasts are small, you can examine them lying down or in the shower.

If they are medium to large, you should examine them lying down. This position spreads your breast as thinly as possible, which makes you more likely to detect a lump, even a very small one.

Let's begin with your *right* breast.

The lying-down position: First, lie on your left side with your knees bent. Now, roll back so that your shoulders are flat on the bed — but don't move your legs. Put your right arm under your head.

If your breasts are very large, place a pillow under your right shoulder.

Your breast is now spread as flat as possible.

The standing position: If you are small-breasted, you can do BSE in the shower, using soap to help your fingers slide easily over your skin.

To examine your right breast stand with your right arm behind your head (Fig. 10.1a).

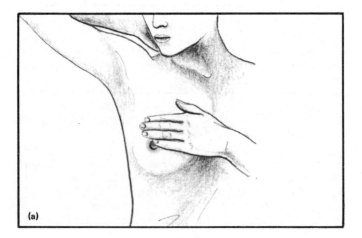

(a)

Step 3: Starting your BSE   You examine all the breast area following an imaginary line of vertical 'strips' starting in your armpit and working up and down across your breast.

You use the flat part of your fingers including the sensitive finger pads. You work in small circles about 5 centimetres across. Use the diagram shown in Figure 10.1b to practise.

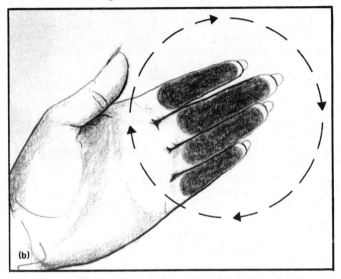

At *each* spot you touch, you should use *two pressures* — *lightly* and then *firmly*.

Feel lightly: With your fingers together and flat, make the first circle with a light pressure, firm enough to make a slight 'dent' in your skin (see Figure 10.1c).

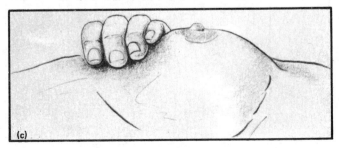

You are feeling for anything near the surface of your skin. *Feel firmly:* At the *same* spot, make a second circle pressing quite firmly, so you can feel any lump *deep* in your breast. Press as firmly as you can without discomfort (Figure 10.1d). Most women can feel their ribs with this firm pressure.

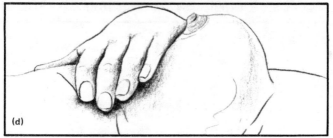

(d)

Now proceed as follows: Using your *left* hand, begin the first 'strip' at your armpit. Make a circle of light, and then of firm pressure at this first spot. Move your hand gradually towards the bra-line, using circles of light and firm pressure at *each* spot.

At the bottom of the bra-line, move across about 2 centimetres to the left and start working upwards to your collar bone, making circles all the time.

Work up and down your breast in strips until you reach your nipple (Fig. 10.1e).

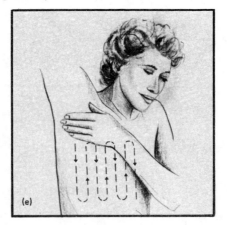

(e)

Step 4: Changing position When you reach the nipple, lie flat on your back. This flattens the inner half of your breast. (If doing BSE in the shower, you don't need to change position).

Complete the nipple strip and continue the circles moving up and down in strips.

Remember the *light and firm pressures* at each spot.

Examine all the breast until you have completed the last strip between your breasts.

Step 5: Checking your armpit Bring your right arm down by your side and feel your armpit firmly. Again you're looking for any lumps.

Now start again, at Step 2, and repeat the procedure for your *left* breast.

Lying down position: Lie on your *right* side, roll back so your shoulders are flat. Put your *left* arm behind your head.

Standing position: Stand with your left arm behind your head. Use your *right* hand to examine your *left* breast.

Regular examinations by a health professional

Many authorities, including the national cancer societies in several countries, recommend that a woman should have a breast examination performed by a trained health professional, at regular intervals. The American Cancer Society, for example, recommended in 1980 that women aged 20 to 40 should have breast examinations at 3-yearly intervals, and from the age of 40 onwards the breast examination should be performed annually. The technique of breast examination used by the trained examiner is identical to that used for breast self examination but the examiner additionally examines the armpit for evidence of enlarged lymph nodes. The recognition of the importance of regular breast examination by health professionals has led to the establishment of 'Breast Clinics' in hospitals or as free-standing clinics in city areas. Many women, mostly from the affluent section of society, are prepared to visit these institutions,but many other women are afraid of going to a hospital or to a special clinic. Their need for breast screening is as great.

Most women do not need to go to a special breast clinic as many family doctors are trained to examine women's breasts, and many women visit their family doctor at least once a year. The woman needs only to ask the family doctor to examine her breasts, or if she prefers, go to a community health clinic and be examined there by a health professional.

It must be said that the effectiveness of breast examination in the detection of breast lumps and their interpretation depends on the skill of the examiner. A recent study shows that some doctors miss or misinterpret breast lumps. This finding and the relative crudeness of breast examination has led some doctors to suggest that an annual breast examination might be replaced by screening by mammography of all women over the age of 40.

Mammography

A mammogram is a special X-ray picture of the breasts, which uses a very low dose of radiation to obtain the picture. Careful investigations have shown that mammography is safe for women over the age of 40 and does not induce cancer even when an annual mammogram is made.

In 1971, a randomized trial of mammography was reported from New York. This trial showed that deaths from breast cancer were reduced among those screened, although some unnecessary operations, including mastectomy, were performed. Later, more carefully organized studies have been reported from Sweden and the Netherlands. These studies show that mammography, using today's techniques, detects breast cancer at an earlier stage than the older methods of mammography.

The studies show that the value of mammography in women over the age of 40 is that it is easy to perform, and that it may detect a breast cancer before it can be detected clinically. The disadvantages of mammography are that a suspicious finding does not necessarily indicate that there is breast cancer. In about ten women in every 1000 examined, the mammogram will detect a suspicious area.

It is important to know that only two suspicious areas in every ten, detected by mammography, turn out to be breast cancer after biopsy.

Current recommendations are that a 'base line' mammogram should be made when the woman is aged about 40 and thereafter every 2 years to the age of 50 and then annually.

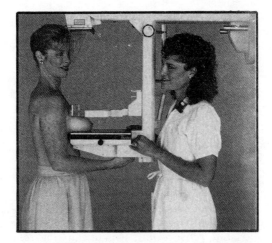

Figure 10.2: A patient and radiographer using a mammography
unit
(Reproduced by kind permission of Laserex Medicon
and Xerox U.K.)

There are certain problems about adopting this advice. At
present, fewer than 25 per cent of women aged 50 ever have a
mammogram, and fewer than 5 per cent have an annual mammogram. If every woman aged 50 or more had a mammogram
each year, the cost would be great and there are insufficient
radiographers to make the picture and insufficient radiolo-
gists to interpret it. As well, a suspicious mammogram means
that further investigations are needed. These usually consist
of an examination of the breast by an experienced doctor and
a biopsy of the suspicious area usually made with a needle.
Some women need to have a minor operation to remove the
suspicious area. The woman usually only needs to remain in
the hospital for a few hours. The doctor makes a small curved
incision along one of the 'tension lines of the breast'. He then
dissects carefully until the area is reached. He then excises it.
Healing is quick and the scar is almost invisible after a few
months.

As these procedures take time and are costly, the problems
mount. Clearly experts and consumers need to discuss the
problems and suggest remedies.

11

THE MENOPAUSE AND THE SKIN

There is no magician's mantle to compare with the skin in its diverse roles of waterproof, overcoat, sunshade, suit of armour and refrigerator, sensitive to the touch of a feather, to temperature and pain, withstanding the wear and tear of three score years and ten, and executing its own running repairs.

So wrote the anatomist R. D. Lockhart in a description that could hardly be bettered.

The skin varies in thickness, being only 0.5 mm thick on the eyelids and 4 mm thick, or more, on the soles of the feet. In places, such as the palms of the hands and the ears, it is firmly bound to the underlying structures. In other places, it is freely moveable. It is smooth or rough, dry or moist, depending on the number of sweat and sebaceous glands it contains. Most of it is covered with hairs, which may be soft and downy, scarcely perceptible, or may be coarse and long. In youth, the skin is firm and elastic; in age it is often loose and wrinkled. It holds a mirror to health and to age, changing in its appearance.

This vital organ, 1.7 square metres in extent, covers the body, protecting and isolating it from the environment. The skin consists of two layers, the outer layer, the epidermis, and the inner layer, the dermis, and both are of equal importance. The epidermis, which interfaces with the environment, is made up of layers of cells all of which are derived from the deepest layer. As the cells mature, they change in shape and in character, until near the surface they lose their nuclei and become a horny layer. From this layer, which varies in thickness, dead cells are constantly shed — over 9 g being lost each day, mostly invisibly, but sometimes embarrassingly as dandruff. This horny layer is vital for life because it is the waterproof layer of the skin. However, certain medications, hormones and poisons can enter the body through the skin, so its waterproofing is not perfect.

The pigmentation of the skin is due to tiny particles of a substance called melanin in the deepest layers of the epidermis. The more melanin, the darker the skin. Melanin protects the skin against the damaging effects of sunlight, which is why 'white'-skinned people tan when exposed to sunlight, but, unfortunately, the skin itself may be damaged, although the tissues beneath it are protected.

The dermis is a felted meshwork of fibrous and elastic tissues, which is riveted to the epidermis by projections that stud its surface (Fig. 11.1). The fibrous tissue is mainly formed from a protein called collagen. In the dermis are found the roots of the hairs, with their accompanying sebaceous glands and the sweat glands, all of which open on the skin's surface through narrow tubes.

The skin is a restless organ, constantly rearranging itself, constantly shedding surface cells and making new cells. Through it hairs grow, which increase in length, live for about 2 years and are then replaced by new hairs growing from the hair follicle deep in the dermis. The sebaceous glands are constantly active, secreting the oil-like sebum, which is similar to the lanolin of sheep's wool, and which greases the surface of the body, keeping the skin pliable. If the gland making sebum becomes blocked, a whitehead, a blackhead or a small cyst will result.

With the passage of the years, and the assaults of the environment, the appearance of the skin changes. The epidermis becomes thinner, drier and may become flaky, particularly in cold climates in winter. The legs are often affected and the flakiness is aggravated by overheated houses in which the relative humidity is low. The reason for the increased rate of shedding of the outer cells of the skin is not understood, but may be related to a reduction in the thickness of the skin with age, and in very old people the skin may become parchment-like and almost transparent.

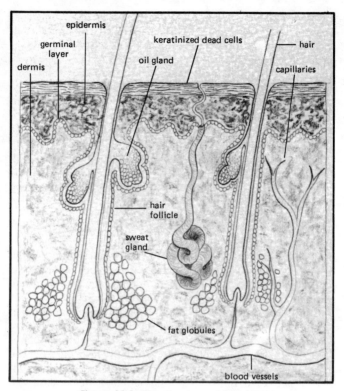

epidermis

germinal layer

keratinized dead cells

hair

dermis

oil gland

capillaries

hair follicle

sweat gland

fat globules

blood vessels

Figure 11.1: The structure of the skin

As a person grows older, the melanin granules, which respond to sunlight by multiplying, become fewer and respond less efficiently, so that skin cancer is likely to become more common.

The dermis also changes as a person ages. It provides support for the tissues lying above and below it and is responsible for the resilience and elasticity of the skin. As a person grows older, a change occurs in the superficial part of the dermis — the elastic fibres become shorter and the meshwork becomes discontinuous.

As well, an alteration occurs in the amount and the integrity of the second type of fibre in the skin, the collagen fibres. The effect of these changes, which begin at about the age of 30, is that fine wrinkles and lines appear on the skin exposed to the sunlight, and the skin under the chin and on the upper arms and legs may become lax and stretched.

The collagen fibres seem to be the most important supporting fibres. The quantity of collagen in the skin is thought to be related to the 'quality' of the skin. The less collagen there is, the fewer elastic fibres are present and the more likely are wrinkles to be found. It has been shown that, from the age of 30, the amount of collagen in the skin decreases by about 1 per cent each year. It decreases rather more rapidly in women than in men, and it is believed that testosterone, the male hormone, protects a man's skin.

Ageing in the exposed skin is influenced considerably by climatic factors, particularly exposure to the sun's ultraviolet light. Ultraviolet light, over a period of time, damages the tissues, causing a break-up of collagen and elastic fibres. The degree to which the sun damages the skin depends on the person's heredity. It occurs less frequently in black races, whose skin is protected by the greater amount of melanin in it, and in certain families of white races.

The changes in the non-exposed parts of the skin are due, mainly, to the alteration in content and distribution of collagen and to a loss of water from the cells that make up the skin. This makes the skin loose and 'saggy'.

The changes in skin have been described at some length as many women attribute the changes in the skin to the menopause. It is certain that this is not so.

Most women in our society would prefer to remain slim, beautiful, with good skin, few wrinkles and glistening hair, well into middle-age.

In this situation, it was to be expected that someone would suggest that hormones might be involved; after all, menopausal women tend to have some wrinkles and as the woman moves into the menopausal years, the wrinkles tend to increase. As oestrogen levels in the blood fall after the menopause, when wrinkles increase, is it not likely that the two findings are connected?

OESTROGEN AND THE SKIN

Does oestrogen improve the quality of the skin and prevent wrinkles?

The evidence that oestrogen increases the thickness of the skin, and makes it more youthful, is confused. A group of doctors in Finland and another in Britain have claimed that oestrogen has this effect. However, a comparable study carried out by another group of doctors in England failed to find that oestrogen, either as tablets or as a skin cream, prevented wrinkles. However, oestrogen may make them less obvious in three ways. First, oestrogen reduces the rate of collagen loss from the skin. Second, oestrogen increases the water content of the skin. Third, it may improve blood flow through the blood vessels in the dermis, which would have the effect of increasing the fluid retained in the skin. The three changes induced by oestrogen would prevent the skin from becoming thin and would tend to make wrinkles less obvious.

If oestrogen treatment does not make much difference to a menopausal woman's skin, is there anything that she can do? Clearly she cannot reverse the changes that have occurred, but she can improve the dry skin that becomes common as a woman grows older.

Cosmetic manufacturers have noted the concern of many women about their skins and offer a bewildering range of 'skin foods', lotions and creams that 'moisturize' dry skin and keep it youthful.

'Skin foods' perhaps have the largest impact. Large numbers of women, persuaded by skilled advertising, purchase creams, lotions, skin tonics and hormone preparations to delay the ageing process in the skin. The products are lavishly launched, superbly packaged, seductively perfumed, and are often very expensive. Do they do what they purport to do; namely, delay the inevitable changes that occur in the skin as a woman ages? The answer is that they do not. The best way to keep the skin in good condition is by cleaning it regularly using soap and water and drying it carefully. There is no cosmetic that will keep a woman's skin youthful if her genetic inheritance decrees that it ages quickly. The skin may be abused in youth by excessive sunbathing, which will hurry the ageing process (and may also cause skin cancer), but it is

Table 11.1: Moisturizers

For a light lotion:
    100 g sorbolene (with 10 per cent glycerine)
    500 ml of hot water
    (0.6 g benzoic acid if required)
    1.5–2.0 ml of perfume essence (if required)

For a heavy lotion/light cream:
    100 g sorbolene (with 10 per cent glycerine)
    300 ml of hot water
    (0.4 g benzoic acid if required)
    1.5–2.0 ml perfume essence (if required)

For a mousse-type cream:
    100 g sorbolene (with 10 per cent glycerine)
    150 ml of hot water
    (0.25 g benzoic acid if required)
    1.5–2.0 ml perfume essence (if required)

For a heavier cream:
    100 g sorbolene (with 10 per cent glycerine)
    100 ml of hot water
    (0.2 g benzoic acid if required)
    1.5–2.0 ml perfume essence (if required)

Courtesy of the Australian Consumers' Association

unlikely that the moisturizing creams that are purchased to limit the effects of that abuse are of any more benefit than the use of a cheap vaseline or lanolin product. Vasoline or lanolin will help the skin to look smooth and soft, and are just as effective as a more expensive moisturizer.

Moisturizers help dry skin, but the effectiveness of the moisturizer bears no relationship to its cost, according to a survey made by the Australian Consumers' Association, (ACA) after studying 72 cosmetic products. The survey showed that there was no relationship between the effectiveness of the product, the user's age, the climatic conditions or the user's skin type. According to the ACA this means that you waste money if you buy a moisturizer that is especially expensive, or said to be for 'mature skin', or for special weathers or seasons, or especially for 'combination' skin, unless you want to indulge yourself or give yourself a 'lift'. Nor are night creams any more effective than other moisturizers.

The survey confirmed that an effective moisturizer used

night and morning after thorough cleansing of the face improves the condition of the skin for about 6 weeks and then maintains its condition.

A commercial skin moisturizer can be bought but it is much cheaper to make one at home. The Australian Consumers' Association (ACA) offers do-it-yourself moisturizers, which prove as effective as any of the commercial products (Table 11.1). ACA found that sorbolene with glycerine (and perfume if desired) is as effective as any of the commercial preparations and is considerably cheaper. Sorbolene (ceto-macrogol cream) is a basic non-prescription skin cream, which many dermatologists recommend to patients who are allergic to perfume. Basically it consists of 10 per cent propylene glycerol (a moistener), 15 per cent of a non-ionic emulsifier (and 0.1 per cent preservative if required), made up in water.

Sorbolene with 10 per cent added glycerine makes a pleasant hand lotion, and it is recommended by ACA as a moisturizer, when made up in the following way. 'The basic method is simple. The sorbolene containing 10 per cent added glycerine (and benzoic acid dissolved in alcohol, only if required as a preservative) is placed in a bowl, and about 100 ml of the hot water added (distilled water may be used if preferred). The mixture is beaten with an old-fashioned egg-beater (we found this better than a processor). The rest of the hot water is added and the mixture beaten again. Perfume essence, if required, can be beaten into the mixture after it has cooled.' The quantities to be used are given in Table 11.1. The moisturizer should be stored in screw-top containers in the fridge, and small quantities removed as needed. An alternative way of preserving the cream is to add benzoic acid dissolved in alcohol (which will need to be made up by a pharmacist). If boiled or distilled water is used to make the lotion, the chance of contamination by bacteria is reduced.

OESTROGEN AND THE HAIR

Does oestrogen improve the quality of the hair?

Growth of hair on the body, in both men and women, depends on the blood levels of a special form of the male hormone, testosterone. A few men lack the enzyme that converts testosterone into this special form and they have hairless bodies. Oestrogen tends to reduce hair growth, but does not influence its quality or quantity. There is no evidence that if oestrogen is given to menopausal women, they will have glistening, healthy hair.

12

THE MENOPAUSE AND THE MIND

There is a belief by many women and many doctors that the menopause is associated with a deterioration in a woman's mental capacity, her ability to reason and to make deductions, and her feeling of 'well being'. Some doctors claim, based on limited experience, that many menopausal women complain of fatigue, depression, nervousness, headaches, irritability, palpitations and poor concentration. While this may be true, the symptoms are likely to be encountered at all ages and by both sexes, so that they cannot be part of the 'menopausal syndrome'. This statement is borne out by several studies. For example, one measure of the degree of psychiatric problems occurring in the years around the menopause is the frequency of first admissions to psychiatric hospitals. In Figure 12.1 it can be seen that fewer first admissions occurred to women aged between 45 and 54, than to those aged between 20 and 24, 25 and 34 and 35 and 44.

The myth that a woman becomes less stable psychologically in her menopausal years has other, more sinister implications. Those people who subscribe to this belief, either consciously or unconsciously, are diminishing women as a sex. If a menopausal woman is believed to be less efficient and have a reduced intellectual capacity, it can be argued that she should not be given an equal opportunity to compete with a man for a job or for promotion to a higher level. If the woman is not in the work force but has chosen to make her home her career, the believed deterioration in her mental balance and capacity may diminish her value as a person in the mind of her husband and family.

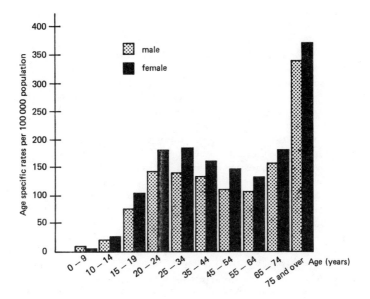

Figure 12.1: Rates of first admission to mental hospitals at various ages (Mental Health Enquiry for England, 1977)

What is the truth of the matter? Are mental problems such as depression, anxiety and reduced mental efficiency more common in the menopausal years?

A problem in answering this question is that studies to investigate the mental state of menopausal women have been poorly designed and often have asked the wrong questions.

For many years psychiatrists diagnosed a supposed mental disease that occurred during the menopausal years, which they called 'involutional melancholia'. It was defined by the American Psychiatric Association in 1968 as:

> . . . a disorder occurring in the involutional period and characterized by worry, anxiety, agitation, and severe insomnia. Feelings of guilt and somatic preoccupations are frequently present and may be of delusional proportions. This disorder is distinguishable from manic depressive illness by the absence of previous episodes . . . and it is distinguishable

from psychotic depressive reaction in that the depression is not due to some life experience.

If this mental illness were real, this would fit in with a knowledge that more women than men, at all ages, presented to doctors and were diagnosed as having depression or anxiety states. It would also fit in with the clinical observation, by some doctors, that the menopausal period was associated with an increase in depression and anxiety.

The question is: 'Are more women depressed in their menopausal years than at other ages?' A major problem in answering the question is that depression occurs at all stages of life, at least after childhood. A survey carried out in Britain in 1980 of over 10 000 women showed that 8 out of 10 had had symptoms of depression at some time of their life; and at the time of the survey, 14 per cent were clinically depressed. Age did not seem to affect the prevalence of depression.

The survey and most others rely on a questionnaire. There are many of these, and they may give different results when administered to the same person.

One questionnaire that is used often is the General Health Questionnaire (GHQ). The version of the GHQ used to determine psychological well-being, or reduction in well-being, is based on 12 questions. The questions related to:

- inability to concentrate
- sleeplessness because of worry
- feeling of no use
- inability to make decisions
- constant strain
- inability to overcome difficulties
- no enjoyment of daily activities
- inability to face problems
- unhappiness and depression
- loss of confidence
- a feeling of worthlessness
- a feeling that everything considered resulted in unhappiness

Nearly 4000 Australian women were asked these questions in a recent survey. The women were chosen so that they were representative of the whole population. A score of 4 or more on the GHQ indicated a high or a severe psychological disturbance. A score of 2 or 3 indicated a moderate psychological disturbance. The study found that 16 per cent of Australian women had a severe psychological disturbance, 14 per cent were moderately or mildly disturbed, and 70 per cent had no psychological problems. Women in the menopausal years (aged 45 to 54) were no more psychologically disturbed than younger or older women.

Similar surveys in the USA, of 400 women, in Britain of 600 women and in Sweden of 900 women, confirm this last finding. In the Swedish study, more detailed questions were asked of women aged 38 to 54. Twenty per cent of the women complained of mental health problems (most often depression or anxiety) that affected their functioning. However, there was no increase in the proportion of women with a mental health problem in or after the menopause compared with younger women. Women who had a mental health problem before the menopause were likely to continue to have the problem after the menopause; however, the main cause of depression and anxiety were life-events. Usually, these were problems with the woman's relationship with her husband or children.

The issue is made more confusing as many depressed women present to a doctor with bodily symptoms rather than psychological symptoms. A study in Britain found that, of women who were identified as depressed, one-third complained of headaches, 29 per cent had 'palpitations' and about 10 per cent complained of abdominal pain. Nearly half of the people complained of three or more symptoms.

These bodily symptoms are often complained of by menopausal women, but are no more common in the menopausal years than in earlier or later ages.

All these studies confirm that there is no disease called involutional melancholia; and that depression is not more common in the menopausal years and cannot be attributed to the hormonal changes occurring at this time.

Despite these findings, some doctors continue to believe that the menopause affects the mental state of women in other ways. They suggest that in the menopausal years, a woman's memory is less effective; her concentration diminishes; she has increased difficulty in making decisions and loses her confidence. In addition it is claimed that a menopausal woman's attention span is reduced, as is her 'reaction time' in response

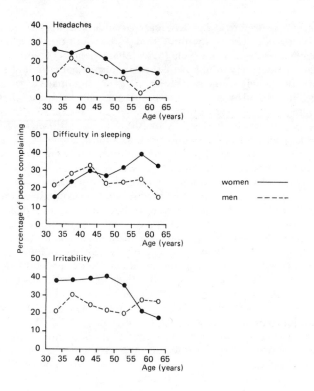

Figure 12.2: Percentage of women and men reporting headaches, difficulty in sleeping and irritability at various ages

to a question. If these observations are true, a menopausal woman may be presumed to be mentally 'inferior' to a younger woman and to men of all ages.

But, are these observations true? In a British study in Oxfordshire, women and men, whose ages varied from 30 to 65, were asked a series of questions about their physical and mental health. The results were plotted for each sex and each age group (at 5 year intervals). When the psychological complaints were analysed in this way some interesting findings emerged. More women had headaches than men, but the percentage of women complaining of headaches declined from about 25 per cent in the 30 to 40 age group to 15 per cent after the age of 50. Difficulty in sleeping increased from the age of 30 in women, peaking at the age of 60, when 40 per cent of women complained. In the case of men, sleeping difficulties declined from a peak of 30 per cent at the age of 40 to 45, to 20 per cent at the age of 50 or more. More women (40 per cent) than men (25 per cent) complained of being irritable. In women the proportion complaining remained steady to the age of 40 to 50 and then declined quite rapidly, so that, by the age of 55, the proportion was similar to that of men aged 55.

From this it is clear that irritability, sleeping difficulties and headaches are not menopausal symptoms (Fig. 12.2).

It has been suggested that 'difficulty in making decisions' and 'loss in confidence' are more common in women than in men and peak after the menopause. The Oxfordshire study investigated these questions. The investigators found that at all ages from 30–35 to 60–65 women did admit to having more difficulty in making decisions than men, and also more had a loss in confidence.

When these complaints were related to the age of the woman 'difficulty in making decisions' peaked in the age group 45 to 50, at 35 per cent, and then declined from the age of 50. After the age of 55 the proportion of women complaining was 20 per cent, the same as in women aged 30 to 45. The complaint of loss of confidence showed a similar pattern (Fig. 12.3).

Another approach was suggested when it became clear that the level of oestrogen in a woman's blood, and presumably her brain, decreased after the menopause. Could it be that the lack of oestrogen influenced her mental well-being? It was

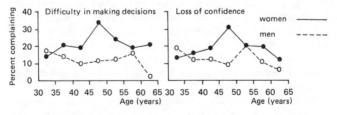

Figure 12.3: Mental ability of men and women at various ages, as measured by the difficulty in making decisions and loss of confidence

believed that oestrogen treatment tended to increase the level in the blood of a substance called 5-hydroxytryptamine. It had been shown in one study that low levels in the blood of this substance was found in many depressed people, so that oestrogen treatment might be effective in relieving depression by increasing the level of 5-hydroxytryptamine in the blood. One study showed that oestrogen had this effect, but subsequent studies failed to find any relationship between the level of 5-hydroxytryptamine and depression, or that oestrogen produced any benefit.

Despite this, some doctors observed that oestrogen given to menopausal women seemed to have a 'mental tonic effect'. A study made in Poland seemed to confirm this observation but the numbers of women investigated were small. A second larger study made in Belgium of menopausal nuns living in a closed convent, who were given either oestrogen tablets or an identical inert pill, failed to find any difference in memory or in any of the other psychological tests used to measure 'mental capacity'.

It seems unlikely that oestrogen has any direct effect as a 'mental tonic', but by relieving the oestrogen-dependent menopausal symptoms of hot flushes, night sweats, insomnia and a painful vagina it could also make the women feel better.

It is still necessary to explain why most of the psychological symptoms attributed to the menopause occur in the 5-year period before menstruation ceases, particularly if menstruation is irregular. At this time the blood levels of oestrogen are fluctuating more widely than in earlier years. It may be that *fluctuating* levels of oestrogen affect mood. Some evidence for this is obtained from studies of women with the premenstrual syndrome. One treatment, which is moderately effective, is to implant oestrogen tablets beneath the woman's skin. The effect of this is to obtain a steady level of oestrogen in the blood.

More research is needed to determine if oestrogen really has a 'mental tonic' effect.

Other attempts have been made to find out if oestrogen impaired a woman's feeling of well-being and her memory when she had no hot flushes. The results are inconclusive. The problem of obtaining an answer to the question is great, as so many things affect a woman during the period of the investigation and these may affect how she feels.

INSOMNIA

Insomnia seems to be more common during the menopausal years than earlier in a woman's life. During the time the woman is having 'hot flushes', insomnia may follow a nocturnal hot flush and its accompanying sweat. If hormone replacement treatment is given, the hot flushes and insomnia cease.

Women who do not have nocturnal hot flushes may find that they are unable to sleep, or that they keep waking up during the night. Sleep may be disturbed because of emotional upset, or unfamiliar surroundings, or because of pain or feelings of depression. Drugs may also cause insomnia, such as some medications or excessive amounts of coffee or tea taken in the evening. It is important to realize, however, that there is no fixed 'normal' amount of sleep. Some people need 10 hours of sleep at night, others feel and perform well on 3 hours. In general, as people grow older they need less sleep and wake more frequently during the night. Older people often 'catnap' during the day, or doze in a chair in the evening. A person's perception of how much he or she sleeps may be inaccurate, and careful studies have shown that a person may be convinced that he or she has not slept all night, when in fact there have been long periods of sleep. Lack of sleep is not a problem in itself and will not in itself affect a person's health — the important thing is to discover what has produced the insomnia and then correct it.

Different people have different patterns of insomnia. For example, some people find it difficult to go to sleep but once they are asleep have no problems. Other people go to sleep easily but wake up early, feeling unconfortable. Other people wake in the middle of the night for long periods.

How can insomnia be managed? Far too many people resort to sleeping pills, which become less effective after a time so that the dose is increased. Sleeping pills (or hypnotics) are useful for brief periods to restore 'normal' patterns of sleep, but if they are taken for longer periods and then stopped, a 'withdrawal' period follows, which may last for up to 3 weeks, during which marked insomnia occurs. The type of hypnotic that should be taken depends on the pattern of insomnia. Barbiturates are no longer commonly prescribed and most doctors prefer to prescribe short-acting benzodiazepines (which are eliminated rapidly from the body) such as temazepam (Euhypnos, Normison), flunitrazepam (Rohypnol), or nitrazepam (Mogadon, Dormicum).

A woman with insomnia should change some habits that interfere with sleep (Table 12.1). If she does this she may not need to take sleeping pills.

Table 12.1: How to help you sleep at night

* Avoid dozing during the day
* Avoid stimulants such as tea or coffee in the late evening
* Avoid alcohol beverages in the late evening
* Alcohol is a sedative and may help you to fall asleep but you may find that you wake up early in the morning
* If you find that a glass of warm milk helps you relax, then take it
* Try to deal with any problems during the day
* Spend at least one hour before going to bed, relaxing and becoming calm
* Remember that insomnia is not a disease in itself; it is the result of something else that should be treated first. Sleeping pills taken for *short periods* help to tide you over while your doctor finds out the cause of your insomnia. But if you take them for longer periods, you will find that they only help you sleep if you increase the dose, and after a while you may find it hard to give them up. If you have been taking sleeping pills for a long time, you will need to give them up, and you must realize that you may get 'withdrawal' symptoms (particularly insomnia), which can go on for weeks.

13

THE MENOPAUSE AND SEXUALITY

Perhaps the most useful statement about sexuality during the menopausal years is that although some women show a decline in their sexual desire, and in their sexual activity and sexual response with advancing age, the sexual response of an individual is unpredictable and a great variation occurs between individuals.

The human sexual response has two main parts. The first is sexual desire or sexual interest. It means that a person is sexually attracted to another person and may or may not attempt to make closer contact. If she or he does, he or she expects to become sexually aroused, in other words, has entered the second part of the sexual response. Sexual arousal may lead to sexual intercourse, to oral sex or to digital sex and, when continued, usually is climaxed by orgasm.

The frequency of sexual intercourse or of orgasm is usually taken as the measure of sexual response, but there are obvious problems in using either of these. For example, some women (and fewer men) only reach orgasm occasionally or never. As well, the ability to reach orgasm may change in frequency at different times. If the woman believes that the man should always initiate sex, the frequency of sexual intercourse may fall because the man has lost interest or appears to have lost interest.

In a study made in Sweden, about 21 per cent of women investigated had an absent or weak interest in sex after the age of 35. By the age of 54, the proportion having a weak sexual interest had increased to 52 per cent. Another Swedish investigation confirmed the finding that a woman's sexual desire tended to decline as she grew older. Out of 3000 women born in 1921, 900 were selected at random. They were interviewed when they were aged 61 to 63. One in every three said that she had lost her interest in sexual relationships.

These studies also suggested that certain women were more likely to have continued sexual interest and enjoyment into old age:

- Women who enjoyed sex in their younger years tended to enjoy sex during their menopausal years.
- Women who had better education, were of a higher social class and were more independent, enjoyed sex more than women of working class backgrounds. A reason for this difference may be that the working class woman had devoted her energies to looking after the home and to rearing the family. Her expectation of sexual enjoyment may have been small, particularly if her husband did not feel it his responsibility to arouse the woman sexually. It is possible that some of the women believed the myth that the sexual response either slows down or ceases when a woman reaches the menopause. It is also possible that better educated women felt more comfortable in telling a man about their sexual needs and helping him understand how he may meet them.
- Women who had episodes of depression during their reproductive years, and had a low self-esteem, were more likely to be less sexually interested or responsive in the menopausal years.
- Women who believed that their sexual role is one of relative passivity may experience a decline in their sexuality because they lack a man's opportunity to experience a sexual encounter.
- The husband's sexual response was a factor that must be considered. If the man were less sexually interested and had less sexual arousal, it is likely that the woman would experience sex less. The decline noted in the menopausal years may be as much to do with the husband's diminished interest as with the wife's.

These findings suggest that the sexual response during the menopausal years is mediated by social or psychological events rather than being dependent on the hormonal changes occurring at that time. Nevertheless, a number of doctors believe that a woman's declining sexual response is dependent on the lack of hormones, particularly the sex hormones oestrogen and androgen (testosterone). It is true that if a woman has severe hot flushes with associated sweating, she is less likely to want sex.

It is also true that if she has a painful dry vagina, sexual intercourse may be unpleasant or painful and avoided. Oestrogen treatment will improve the woman's sex life by relieving these symptoms, but the improvement is not due to a direct effect of oestrogen on the woman's sexual desire or her sexual arousal. In laboratory animals, a lack of the male sex hormone, androgen (testosterone), is associated with a decreased sexual response. This is also true in a few aged males, when a low blood level of testosterone is associated with erectile failure. But there is no evidence that menopausal women need testosterone to retain sexual arousal (libido). The results of reported investigations (made since 1975) are contradictory, but the concensus is that the administration of testosterone (usually as an injection) has no proved beneficial effect in improving a menopausal woman's sexual response.

HOW TO IMPROVE SEXUAL RELATIONSHIPS

The sexual problems that affect women during and after the menopause are no different from those affecting younger women, with one exception. This is the problem of painful intercourse. Painful intercourse may occur at all ages for a variety of reasons, but in menopausal and postmenopausal women it may be due to a lack of oestrogen. Oestrogen lack leads to a thinner vaginal lining, to a burning pain or discomfort in the vagina and to painful intercourse. The treatment is to give oestrogen, as was discussed on page 46.

However, it may be important for the couple to explore the relationship as well.

Lack of sexual desire, lack of sexual arousal and failure to reach orgasm are due, usually, to conflict in the couple's relationships. The underlying factors may be that the couple have stopped talking to each other, and that neither partner is able to tell the other of her or his sexual needs or feelings. The woman may see her husband as fat, ageing or drinking too much. He may see her body as flabby and ageing and may compare it adversely with those of the models and actresses he sees on television. The woman may sense this and lose her confidence, becoming depressed. She may no longer feel she has any worth to her husband. She may have become bored with the way her husband makes love, particularly if she has been brought up to believe that the man is always the initiator.

The first way to improve matters is for the couple to try to talk to each other about their relationship. It may help if first they both have a medical check-up to make sure that the problem is not an underlying undiscovered illness. If the woman is able to talk about her sexual desires, her needs and her feelings, and her husband is able to reciprocate, the problem may be resolved. If they always make love in exactly the same way, they may agree to try something more innovative. If the man believes that unless his wife reaches orgasm while he thrusts inside her she is frigid, he needs to reassess this belief. It is wrong. Fewer than half of all women reach orgasm in this way. To help his wife reach orgasm, she may ask her partner to stimulate her clitoris, at her direction, or she may find she reaches orgasm by masturbating.

The second way to improve her sexual enjoyment is for her to seek sexual counselling from a doctor or a psychiatrist and to induce her husband to come with her for some of the sessions at least.

Sexuality includes cuddling, touching and holding as well as sexual intercourse. Sexuality includes feeling that you are of value to your partner and he values you. And this is of considerable importance to a woman in her menopausal years.

BIBLIOGRAPHY

In this bibliography we have only given key references, which readers might care to obtain if they wish for further information.

Chapter 1   INTRODUCTION

(page 2)
McKinlay S and McKinlay J, 'Selected Studies of the Menopause', *J. Biosocial Sci.*, 1973, 5, 533–55; Colombat de L'Isère, 'Hygiene Rules Relative to the Menopause', quoted by Ricci J V, *One Hundred Years of Gynecology*, Philadelphia, Blakeston, 1945.

(page 2)
Women's attitudes to the menopause in the USA:
Lieblum S and Swartzman L C, *Maturitas*, 1986, 8, 47–56.

Chapter 2   A WOMAN'S REPRODUCTIVE ORGANS and
Chapter 3   MENSTRUATION AND THE MENOPAUSE

The anatomy and physiology of the genital tract
Described in Llewellyn-Jones D, *Fundamentals of Obstetrics and Gynaecology*, vol 2: Gynaecology, 4th Edition, London, Faber and Faber, 1986.

Chapter 4 PSYCHOLOGICAL CHANGES DURING THE MENOPAUSE

(pages 22–26)
Life stress and menopausal symptoms
Greene J G and Cooke J, *Brit. J. Psychiatry*, 1986, 136, 486–91; Poht D E and La Rocca S A, 'Social and Psychological Correlates of Menopausal Symptoms', *Psychol. Medicine*, 1980, 42, 335–45.

Chapter 5 THE PHYSICAL SYMPTOMS OF THE MENOPAUSE

(page 29)
Proportion of menopausal women who have 'distressing' symptoms
Thompson B et al., *J. Biosocial Sci.*, 1973, 5, 71–82; James C E, *Brit. J. Obst. and Gynaec.*, 1984, 91, 56–62.
(page 30)
Bungay G J et al. (Oxfordshire Study): *Brit. Med. J.*, 1980, 281, 181–84; (Swedish studies) Person T et al., *Acta Obst. Gynaec. Scand.*, 1983, 62, 289–96; 1984, 63, 257–70; Hagstad A and Jansen P O, *Acta Obst. Gynaec. Scand.*, Supp 134, 1986, 59–65.

Chapter 6 HOW TO MANAGE THE MENOPAUSE

(page 35)
Psychological symptoms — life-stress and its effect on menopausal symptoms
See, for example, Ballinger S E, *Maturitas*, 1985, 7, 315–27.
(page 36)
Physical symptoms: concern about body weight — slimming practices and dieting
Crawford D A and Worsley A, *Med. J. Aust.*, 1988, 148, 325–31.
(page 44)
Liver function and oestrogens
Moore B et al., 'HRT and Liver Function Tests', *Maturitas*, 1987, 9, 7–15; Von Shoultz B, *Acta Obst. Gynaec. Scand.*, 1985, Supp 130, 26.

(page 46)
Transdermal oestrogen
Holst J et al., *Maturitas*, 1987, 9, 63–67.

(page 48)
Oestrogen implants — level of blood oestrogen needs monitoring
Guirgis R R, *Lancet*, 1987, 2, 856 (letter).

(page 50)
Which is the safest progestogen? (1) None better than any other
Tikkanen M J et al., *Maturitas*, 1986, 8, 7–17; Jensen J et al., *Amer. J. Obst. Gynec.*, 1987, 156, 66–71.

(page 50)
(2) Medroxyprogesterone safest
Hirvonen R et al., *New Eng. J. Med.*, 1981, 304, 560.

(page 50)
(3) Medroxyprogesterone less effective in preventing changes in endometrial cells
Lane G et al., *Fert Steril*, 1986, 45, 345–52.

(page 50)
Von Shoultz B, 'Climacteric Complaints as Influenced by Progestogens', *Maturitas*, 1986, 8, 107–12.

(page 52)
Continuous daily oestrogen and progestogen
Staland B, *Maturitas*, 1981, 3, 145–56; Matteson L A et al., *Maturitas*, 1982, 4, 95–102.

(page 53)
Vaginal smears no value
James C E et al., *Brit. J. Obst. Gynaec.*, 1984, 91, 56–62.

(page 54)
Annual endometrial biopsy not needed
Menopause panel discussion, *Amer. J. Obst. Gynec.*, 1987, 156, 1322–25.

(page 55)
Testosterone of benefit
Studd J W W et al., *Brit. J. Obst. Gynaec.*, 1978, 84, 314; Schlyler-Saunders E, 'The Menopausal Syndrome', *Yearbook of Obstetrics and Gynecology*, Greenblat R (ed), New York, 1974.

(page 55)
Testosterone of no value
Dow M G T et al., *Brit. J. Obst. Gynaec.*, 1985, 90, 361–64;
Barlow D H et al., *Obst. Gynec.*, 1986, 67, 321–35.
(page 56)
Clonidine as transdermal preparation
Nagamani M et al., *Amer. J. Obst. Gynec.*, 1987, 156, 561–
65.

Chapter 6   APPENDIX: OESTROGEN METABOLISM

General
Casey M L and MacDonald P, *The Menopause*, Buchsbaum H J
(ed), New York, Springer-Verlag, 1983, 1–23; Fishman J and
Matucci C P, 'New Concepts of Oestrogen Activity', *Meno-
pause and Postmenopause*, Pasetto N (ed), Lancaster,
M.T.P., 1980.

Chapter 7   THE SIDE-EFFECTS OF HORMONAL TREATMENT

(page 60)
Oestrogen and endometrial cancer, general review
Lipshitz S and Bernstein S G, *The Menopause*, Buchsbaum H J
(ed), New York, Springer-Verlag, 1983, 102–29.
(page 62)
Discomfort from endometrial biopsy
Polson A W et al., *Brit. Med. J.*, 1984, 288, 981–83.
(page 62)
Breast cancer and oestrogen replacement
Kaufman D W et al., *J. Amer. Med. Assoc.*, 1984, 252, 63–67.
(page 63)
Cardiovascular disease
Wilson P W et al., *Amer. Cardiol.*, 1980, 46, 649–54.

Chapter 8   A HEALTHY DIET FOR MENOPAUSE AND AFTER

General
Looking Forward to Better Health, vol. 2: *Towards Better
Nutrition for Australia*, Canberra, AGPS, 1987; *Eating
Disorders — the Facts*, Llewellyn-Jones D and Abraham S,
2nd Edition, Sydney, Oxford Univ. Press, 1987.

(page 65)
Slimming practices and dieting
Crawford D A and Worsley A, *Med. J. Aust.*, 1988, 148, 325–31.
(page 70)
Food fibre better than added fibre
Topping D, *Med. J. Aust.*, 1986, 144, 307–9.

Chapter 9   OSTEOPOROSIS

General
'Consensus Conferences', *J. Amer. Med. Ass.*, 1984, 252, 799–802; *Brit. Med. J.*, 1987, 295, 914–15; *Lancet*, 1987, 2, 833–35.
(pages 77–81)
Heany R P and Barger-Lux M J, 'Calcium, Bone Metabolism and Structural Failure', *Triangle*, 1985, 24, 91–100; Arlot M et al., *Brit. Med. J.*, 1984, 289, 577, Riggs B L and Melton I J, *New Eng. J. Med.*, 1986, 314, 1676–86.
(page 83)
Raitz L G, *New Eng. J. Med.*, 1983, 309, 29–35 (notes that vitamin D_3 also reduces bone calcium).
(page 84)
Changes in bone mass with ageing
Riggs B L and Melton I J, *New Eng. J. Med.*, 1986, 314, 1676–86.
(page 84)
Rates of bone loss
Riggs B L and Melton I J, *New Eng. J. Med.*, 1986, 314, 1676–86.
(pages 86–88)
Causes of osteoporosis
Smith R, *Brit. Med. J.*, 1987, 294, 329–32.
(page 87)
Reduced mobility and bone loss
Epstein L, *Lancet*, 1984, 1, 307.
(page 88)
Smoking increases bone loss
Jensen R et al., *New Eng. J. Med.*, 1985, 313, 973–75.

(page 89)
Bone fractures in the elderly
Kiel D J, *New Eng. J. Med.*, 1987, 317, 1169–74.
(page 91)
Calcium intake reduces bone loss in menopausal years
Nordin B E C et al., *Brit. Med. J.*, 1987, 295, 1276–77.
(page 91)
Doubt if calcium intake reduces bone loss
Riis B et al., *New Eng. J. Med.*, 1987, 316, 173–77.
(page 93)
Value of prescribing calcium as well as oestrogen?
(1) Beneficial
Christiansen S et al., *Lancet*, 1985, 2, 800–4; Selby P C and Peacock M, *Lancet* 1985, 2.
(page 93)
(2) Doubtful value
Riis B et al., *Amer. J. Obst. Gynec.*, 1987, 156, 61–65.
(page 93)
Ettinger B et al., 'Postmenopausal Bone Loss Prevented by Treatment with Low-dose Oestrogen', *Ann. Int. Med.*, 1987, 106, 40–48.
(page 94)
Routine X-ray screening of bones to detect osteoporosis and to identify women needing oestrogen
(1) Cost-effective
Nordin B E C et al., *Brit. Med. J.*, 1987, 291, 1276–77.
(page 94)
(2) Not cost effective
Amer. J. Obst. Gynec., 1987, 156, 1352–55.
(page 94)
Oestrogen most effective agent in reducing bone loss
'Consensus Development Conference — Prophylaxis and Treatment of Osteoporosis', *Brit. Med. J.*, 1987, 295, 914–15; Editorial, *Lancet*, 1987, 2, 833–35.
(page 95)
Does exercise reduce bone loss?
Editorial, *J. Amer. Med. Ass.*, 1987, 257, 3115–17; Chow R et al., *Brit. Med. J.*, 1987, 295, 1441–44.
(page 96)
Calcitonin of doubtful value
Hurley D L et al., *New Eng. J. Med.*, 1984, 317, 537–41.

(page 96)
Calcitonin of value
MacIntyre I et al., 'Calcitonin for Prevention of Menopausal Bone Loss', *Lancet*, 1988, 1, 900–2.

Chapter 10   THE MENOPAUSE AND BODY SYSTEMS

(page 98)
Cardiovascular disease. (1) Lipoprotein–cholesterol
Miller V E, *Lancet*, 1984, 1, 263.
(page 99)
(2) Does oestrogen replacement therapy reduce cardiovascular disease in post-menopausal women?
See, for example, Tikkanan M and Nikkila E, *Acta Obst. Gynaec. Scand.*, 1987, Supp. 140, 39–45 (references to earlier papers in the article); Bush T L et al., *Circulation*, 1987, 75, 11023–9); Silferstolpe G and Crona N, *Acta Obst. Gynaec. Scand.*, 1985, Supp. 134, 93–95.
(page 100)
(3) Oestrogen no protection after natural menopause but offers protection after premature (surgical) menopause
Colditz G et al., *New Eng. J. Med.*, 1984, 316, 1105–10.
(page 103)
The breasts. (1) Breast cancer screening
'U.S. Preventive Services Task Force: Recommendations for Breast Cancer Screening', *J. Amer. Med. Ass.*, 1987, 257, 2196–203.
(pages 104–108)
(2) How to perform breast self examination
Material kindly provided by the Anti-Cancer Council of Victoria, Australia.
(pages 109–110)
(3) Mammography a better screening method than BSE or clinical examination
Baker L H, *Ca-A-Cancer*, 1982, 32, 194–230; Veerbek A L M et al., *Lancet*, 1984, 1, 1222–24; Taber L et al., *Lancet*, 1985, 1, 829, 32.

Chapter 11   THE MENOPAUSE AND THE SKIN

(page 116)
Brincat M et al., *Obstetrics and Gynaecology*, 1987, 70, 840–44.

Chapter 12   THE MENOPAUSE AND THE MIND

(pages 122–126)
Mental health in the climacteric
Hallstrom T and Sammelens E, *Acta Obst. Gynaec. Scand.*, 1985, Supp. 130, 13–18; Ballinger C B, *Brit. Med. J.*, 1985, 3, 344–46; Pitt B, *Midlife Crisis*, London, Sheldon Press, 1980; Gath D et al., *Brit. Med. J.*, 1987, 294, 213–18.

Chapter 13   THE MENOPAUSE AND SEXUALITY

(page 131)
Value of testosterone injections (1) Value
Studd W W et al., *Brit. J. Obst. Gynaec.*, 1977, 84, 314–16; Burger H et al., *Brit. Med. J.*, 1987, 1, 936.
(page 131)
(2) No value
Dow M G T, *Brit. J. Obst. Gynaec.*, 1983, 90, 361–66; Sander D and Bancroft J, *J. Clin. Endo. Metabol.*, 1982, 11, 639–59; Bachman H, *Maturitas*, 1985, 7, 211–16.

GLOSSARY

Artificial menopause The cessation of a woman's menstrual period following surgical removal of her ovaries or radiation to her ovaries, and if not treated she may develop menopausal symptoms.

Body mass index (BMI) An index of the body weight to determine if the person is underweight, if weight is in the normal range, or if the person is overweight or obese. The index is calculated using the following formula:

$$\frac{\text{Weight in kilograms}}{\text{Height in metres} \times \text{height in metres}}$$

Cholesterol An important constituent of animal fats (lipids) which is involved in the development of narrowing (atherosis) of the arteries of the heart. In the body, cholesterol links with lipoproteins to be carried in the blood. Cholesterol is linked with several of the lipoprotein fractions, which have different densities. They are named high-density lipoprotein (HDL), low-density lipoprotein (LDL) and very-low-density lipoprotein (VLDL). The higher the level of the LDL–cholesterol fraction in the blood, the greater is the risk of a heart attack.

Climacteric (Sometimes referred to as 'perimenopause') The period of hormonal and psychological adjustment around the time of the menopause. The word is no longer in fashion and menopause is used in its place. If the term 'menopause' is used accurately it means the permanent cessation of menstruation, not the years around the event.

Collagen The white substance that forms fibres in the connective tissues, cartilege and bone. On boiling, it turns into gelatin.

Cortical layer of bone The compressed outer layer of true bone. Also called cortical or compact bone.

Dermis The layer of the skin between the outside layer (the epidermis) and the connective tissue. The dermis contains hair follicles, sweat glands and blood vessels.

Endometrium   The inner layer of the uterus, which contains the uterine glands.

Epidermis   The outer layer of the skin.

Follicle stimulating hormone   One of the hormones secreted by the pituitary gland, which stimulates the growth of a number of egg cells in the ovary each month during a woman's reproductive years. It is also known as FSH. FSH stimulates the cells that surround the egg to secrete oestrogen.

Labia   The 'lips' that surround the entrance to the vagina. The outer lips (labia majora) are filled with fatty tissue and have hair on the outer surface; the inner lips (labia minora) are thin and have no hair on them.

Luteinizing hormone (LH)   The second of the pituitary hormones that are involved in releasing an ovum (egg) each month during the reproductive years. LH then acts on the cell nest from which the egg escaped and converts it into a 'yellow body'. The yellow body (corpus luteum) secretes oestrogen and progesterone.

Mammography   The technique of making an X-ray picture of the breasts; it uses a very small, and safe quantity of radiation. The picture is called a **mammogram**.

Oestrogen   The main female sex hormone.

Osteoporosis   The loss of bone tissue and of calcium, which renders the bone brittle and more likely to fracture.

Perimenopause   *See* Climacteric.

Periosteum   The thin, transparent tissue that covers bone.

Progesterone   The second of the female sex hormones.

Progestogens   Progesterone-like substances produced in a laboratory. In the body they have many of the effects of the natural hormone progesterone, but unlike it, they are effective if taken by mouth.

Quetelet Index   Another name for the body mass index, so called after the scientist who first used it.

Trabecular bone   The inner part of the long bones, and most of the vertebral bones of the spine. It is made up of a complicated honeycomb of bony tissue.

Vulva   A woman's external genitals.

INDEX

anxiety   123
artificial menopause, *see*
   menopause, artificial

biopsy, breast   111
   biopsy, endometrium   54, 61
bleed, withdrawal   51, 52, 61
blood pressure, high   63
BMI, *see* body mass index
body mass index   71–2
bone
   changes with ageing   76,
      85–7
   compact layer, *see* bone,
      cortical
   cortical   79–80, 86
   density measurement   95
   description of   79–81
   dynamism of   78–82
   fractures of   76, 87, 90–91
   remodelling of   81
   spongy layer, *see* bone,
      trabecular
   structure of   79, 81
   trabecular   79, 80, 86
breasts
   cancer, *see* cancer, breast
   changes after menopause   13
   examination of   54, 109–10
   mammography   110–11
   self-examination of   103–9

caffeine intake   41

osteoporosis and, *see*
   osteoporosis, caffeine intake
   and
calcitonin, *see* hormones,
   calcitonin
calcium
   and bone   76, 82–83, 87
   in diet   71, 84, 92–3
   and osteoporosis   92
cancer
   breast   60, 104
   cervix   11
   endometrium   60–2
cardiovascular disease   63, *see*
   also heart disease
   oestrogen and, *see* oestrogen,
      cardiovascular disease and
cervix, uterine
   description   10
   cancer of, *see* cancer, cervix
cholesterol   99–100
civilization, diseases of   43
climacteric   1
collagen, *see* skin, collagen in
cortical bone, *see* bone, cortical

endometrium, cancer of, *see*
   cancer, endometrium
Estigen   43
ethinyl oestradiol   43, 58
exercise   96
   and osteoporosis, *see*
      osteoporosis, exercise and

Fallopian tubes   11–12
fat in diet   66–7
Feminone   43
fibre in diet   68–70
flashes, hot, *see* flushes, hot
fluoride for osteoporosis   96
flushes, hot   31, 55, 56
follicle stimulating hormone, *see* hormones, follicle stimulating
fractures, bone, *see* bone, fractures of
FSH, *see* hormones, follicle stimulating

gall bladder disease   45, 64
General Health Questionnaire   122
genital organs   5–11
    changes in with age   12–13
genitals
    external 5–9
    internal   9–11
Gestrinone   51

hair, oestrogen and   118–19
Harmogen   43
heart disease   98–102
height, decrease in with ageing   76
hip fractures   90
hormonal replacement treatment (therapy)
    contraindications to   55
    investigations before use   53–4
    principles of   54
    side-effects of   60–4
    regimens of   54
hot flushes (flashes), *see* flushes, hot
hormones
    calcitonin   84, 97
    follicle stimulating   15–19
    gonadotrophic releasing   14–15
    luteinizing   15–19
    oestrogen   15, 53, 60–4, 94, 99
    parathyroid   84
    progesterone   12, 17
    progestogens   50, 61, 62, 94, 100
    testosterone   19, 48, 96, 131
hymen   7

implants (of oestrogen), *see* oestrogen, implant of
incontinence, urinary   13, 102–3
insomnia   127–8
'involutional melancholia'   121

Kliogest   43
Kolpon pessaries   43

labia majora, description   5
labia minora, description   6
LH, *see* hormones, luteinizing
life expectancy   21
lipids (in blood)   99–100
lipoproteins   98
luteinizing hormone, *see* hormones, luteinizing
Lynoral   43

mammography   110–11
medroxyprogesterone   50, 54, 56, 100
menopause
    approach to   37
    artificial   4
    attitudes to   2–3, 36
    average age at   3
    breasts and   62–3, 103–9
    coping with   25
    cultural views of   2
    doctors' views of   20–2
    hormonal changes in   19
    management of physical symptoms   40–59

management of psychological symptoms 35–40
menstrual disturbances in 28–9
mental health and 120–4
premature 4
priorities in 37
psychological symptoms of 25
symptoms, frequency of 29
urinary tract and 102–3
Microlut 51
micronized oestrogen, see oestrogen, micronized
Micronor 51
Microval 51
middle age, problems of 37
Mixogen 43
moisturizers 116–18

night sweats 42
norethisterone 51, 56
norgestrel 100

obesity 65, 71–3
oestradiol 43, 58–9
oestriol 59
oestrogen
cancer and 60–2
cardiovascular disease and 99–100
conjugated equine, see oestrogen, equine
equine 42, 43
heart disease and 98–101
injection of 48
implant of 48–9
in menstrual cycle 14–16
metabolism of 57–59
micronized 46, 59
'natural' 42, 43, 44, 45
oral 46
osteoporosis, and 85
side-effects of 45, 60–4
skin and 116–18

synthetic 42, 43
transdermal 43, 46–8
vaginal 46
varieties of 42–51
Ogen 43
osteoporosis
caffeine intake and 87
calcitonin and, see hormones, calcitonin
calcium and 88
causes of 87
costs of 90
definition of 78
exercise and 88
fractures and 78, 90–1
prevention of 88, 92–7
sex hormones and 87, 93–5, 96
smoking and 89
symptoms of 90
treatment of 97
ovaries 12
overweight, see obesity
Ovestrin 43
oviducts, see Fallopian tubes
ovulation 14, 17

Pap smear 40
perimenopause, see climacteric
perineum 8
periosteum 79
Premarin 43
premature menopause, see menopause, premature
Prempak 43
Primolut N 51
progesterone, see hormones, progesterone
progestogens, see also hormones, progestogens
treatment with 51, 52, 56
side-effects of 50, 99
Progynova 43
Provera 51, 56

Quetelet index, *see* body mass index

Relaxation exercises   38–40

sex hormones, *see* hormones
sexual intercourse, painful   33, 131
sexual relations, improving   131
sexual response   129
sexuality and menopause, *see* menopause, sexuality and
skin
  changes in with ageing 113–14
  collagen in   80, 115
  description of   112–114
  'foods'   116
  moisturizers   117
  oestrogens and, *see* oestrogen, skin and
sleeping pills   127
smoking   41, 87
sugar in diet   68
sweats   42

testosterone, *see* hormones, testosterone

thrombosis, venous   45, 63
trabecular bone, *see* bone, trabecular
transdermal oestrogen, *see* oestrogen, transdermal

urinary incontinence, *see* incontinence, urinary
uterine cervix, *see* cervix, uterine
Uterogestan   51
uterus, description   10

vagina   9
vaginal oestrogen   46
vaginal smears   53
vaginal symptoms
  burning   33
  discomfort   33
  pain   33, 131
venous thrombosis, *see* thrombosis, venous
vitamins in diet   71
vitamin D_3 84, 96

withdrawal bleed, *see* bleed, withdrawal